Advance Praise for *Positive Parenting*

"For those who have not yet had the experiences of being a parent, a book such as Dr. Eden's that takes a practical, easy to remember, common sense approach to the subject is a must."
— James A. Stockman III, M.D.
   President, American Board of Pediatrics

"Dr. Eden's *Positive Parenting* remains a must-have book for every parent's night table. His wealth of knowledge and experience are always evident but it is his positive, upbeat and supportive approach that has the power to calm even the most frazzled parent's nerves. His credo, 'Relax and enjoy your baby' resonates from generation to generation."
— David Katzner
   President, The National Parenting Center

"Dr. Alvin Eden exudes experience—nearly fifty years as a pediatrician—addressing the health, sickness and development of children. His insights and advice reflect deep wisdom and common sense while maintaining an up to date awareness of the latest information for raising healthy happy children."
— Lawrence Diller, M.D.
   Author of *Running on Ritalin* and *The Last Normal Child*

"Every pediatrician and every parent should have a copy of this book."
— Donald Gribetz, M.D.
   Professor Emeritus of Pediatrics, Mount Sinai School of Medicine

"Dr. Alvin Eden brings his many decades of extensive clinical experience as a pediatrician to this book."
— Philip Lanzkowsky, M.D.
   Executive Director and Chief-of-Staff, Schneider Children's Hospital

"This book provides thoughtful, well-researched, and useful information for new parents. The author has a great deal of experience caring for children (and their parents), and he applies that experience by providing common sense advice with humor and clarity. Even experienced parents will benefit from the wisdom and balance Dr. Eden provides. Most importantly, the book lives up to the title by describing the many ways in which a positive and encouraging approach can enhance the early lives of children, for the baby and the parents."
— Julia McMillan, M.D.
   Professor of Pediatrics, Johns Hopkins School of Medicine

"Dr. Alvin Eden's advice to parents is practical and helpful. *Positive Parenting* is filled with common sense, humor, and wisdom."
— H. Garry Gardner, M.D., FAAP

Positive
Parenting

Hatherleigh Press

5-22 46th Avenue, Suite 200

Long Island City, NY 11101

www.hatherleighpress.com

Library of Congress Cataloging-in-Publication data available upon request.

ISBN: 978-1-57826-252-6

All Hatherleigh Press Books are available for bulk purchase, special promotions, and premiums. For information about reselling and special purchase opportunities, please call 1-800-528-2550 and ask for the Special Sales Manager.

Cover design by Deborah Miller

Interior design by Allison Furrer

10 9 8 7 6 5 4 3 2 1

Printed in the United States

Positive Parenting

Raising Healthy Children from
Birth to Three Years

ALVIN N. EDEN, M.D.

Foreword by James A. Stockman III, M.D.
President of the American Board of Pediatrics

Improve your life. Change your world.

New York

Dedication

To Elaine
And to our children, Robert and Elizabeth,
and their children in chronological order—
Jonathan, Michael, Geneviève, Alexander,
Michele, and Elizabeth

With Much Love

Special Thanks

*I want to thank Gladys Villalta
for her invaluable secretarial help,
and my editors, Andrea Au and Alyssa Smith,
for their tireless efforts and support.*

Author's Note

As I have stated in all my books, I firmly believe in the equality of the sexes. The English language still does not provide any graceful word to substitute for "his" and "her" or "he" and "she." Therefore, I have again decided to continue to alternate the pronouns used to describe gender, chapter by chapter, starting with the Introduction, thus giving equal time to both sexes. Please remember that these pronouns refer to your child, even if your baby is the opposite sex – except, of course, where I make remarks that apply specifically to boys or girls. I start off the Introduction with "she," a decision made by the flip of a coin.

For similar reasons, "you" will refer to both mother and father, with one exception – the discussion relating to breast feeding.

Table of Contents

Foreword

There are many books on parenting, so many that there is a saying on the subject: "reading a book on good parenting does not make you a good parent any more than standing in the middle of your garage makes you a good car." Believers in this saying may change their mind after a read of Dr. Eden's *Positive Parenting*. True the many insights provided by Dr. Eden may not make for a totally "complete" parenting experience, but they will fill in many of the blanks, even for the most seasoned of parents. There is indeed no better way to learn about parenting than by being a parent. I have been involved with the teaching of residents in training in pediatrics for more than three decades and have worried about those residents who were not parents themselves and the possibility that they were not becoming truly well rounded in their educational experience. For those who have not yet had the experiences of being a parent, a book such as Dr. Eden's that takes a practical, easy to remember, common sense approach to the subject is a must.

One can see in *Positive Parenting* a thoughtful approach to all aspects of child rearing, an approach that addresses the most current thinking on timely issues such as the influence of breastfeeding on child development, including the latest information on its impact relative to behavior and intelligence. While dealing with what's new, Dr. Eden also puts into perspective what has and should remain unchanged in parenting approaches over the years. Yes, our parents, and even grandparents, did do some things right.

When I first picked up *Positive Parenting* I was curious to learn how the word "positive" would be applied to the subject of parenting. While everyone probably knows what negative parenting might be, what might "positive" suggest in this regard? After reading Dr. Eden's book, I then referred to Daniel Webster to see which of his definitions best suited the "positive" in *Positive Parenting*. Bet you were not aware that there are more than 20 somewhat different meanings of the word positive. Two, however, most appropriately apply to the approaches chosen by Dr. Eden. They are "capable of being constructively applied" and "charged with electricity." Both definitions describe *Positive Parenting*. You can take the information learned and constructively apply the learnings at home. You will be charged with electricity while doing so!

— James A. Stockman III, M.D.
  President, American Board of Pediatrics

Introduction

The first edition of *Positive Parenting* was published in 1980 and happily was a big success. The reviews were excellent and the feedback from the readership was so good that it almost gave me a swelled head. What came across loud and clear was that new parents found it easy to read, easy to understand, full of true and sometimes funny anecdotes, and most important, it made parenting less worrisome and more enjoyable. As one of my patients said to me, "You know, Dr. Eden, it sounds just like you talking to me. I always feel better when I leave your office."

So why have I revised and updated *Positive Parenting* now? First of all, the 1980 edition is out of print and unavailable to an entirely new generation of first-time parents. Secondly, a whole lot has changed in the parenting business since then. Let me give you a few examples: We now know much more about how to raise a child's I.Q., how to help prevent Sudden Infant Death Syndrome (SIDS), and the dangers from the misuse of antibiotics. We have new approaches to the prevention of childhood obesity and type II diabetes. The dangers of iron deficiency and its association with increased lead absorption have been established. We now know a great deal more about the problems of day-care, single-parent households and mothers going back to work early. These are just a few of the many topics now included or expanded on in this new edition of *Positive Parenting*. The final reason for my decision to re-write and re-publish *Positive Parenting* was the opportunity to finally remove mention of O. J. Simpson, who in 1980 was considered a role model for children from the introduction.

The great challenge of "positive parenting" is to raise a happy, healthy, smart, and emotionally stable child who will grow up to be successful in her career and in her interpersonal relationships. All of us want the very best for our children, but how to achieve that goal is the big question. Although the right set of genes, good luck, and common sense all help, much more is needed to do the very best job. Helping parents nurture their child so that she may reach her full physical, emotional, and intellectual potential is my purpose in writing this book. That is indeed a tall order, and who am I to undertake it?

I have been a practicing pediatrician for over forty years as well as a father and grandfather. These roles have given me abundant experience with infants and children. I have had the opportunity to observe literally thousands of parents and children in action, and have been in the child-rearing profession long enough to come to some definite conclusions. There are right ways and wrong ways to raise children. Knowing what not to do is just as important as knowing what to do. All of us make many mistakes along the way, but the bottom line is to be able to realize when we are on the wrong track and to do something constructive about it. Mistakes in child rearing are unavoidable, but repeating the same errors over and over again is not acceptable.

There is no question that the first three years of life are crucial to the intellectual development of your youngster. Unlike all the other organs of the body, the brain is almost fully grown by age three, and so during this critical period of rapid brain growth, it is particularly important not to deprive the brain of essential nutrients, particularly iron, in order to achieve maximum intellectual potential. I.Q. points are essential for success and you can increase your child's I.Q., as well as prevent the loss of I.Q. points, by following my simple suggestions. This will be discussed in detail as we go along.

More and more evidence has accumulated pointing to the fact that future physical and emotional development also rests in large measure on what happens during these first three years. The experiences you give your child from birth to three years will greatly influence her intellectual, physical, and emotional development throughout her lifetime. If these experiences are not provided, the chances of achieving her full potential will be reduced. Let me give an example of this: Two babies are born with equal genetic potential. Baby A is left in her crib most of the time to fend for herself, except for feeding, changing, and bathing. Baby B engages in stimulating play and activities, interacting during much of her waking time with her parents or another primary caregiver. Without question, Baby B will have a tremendous advantage over Baby A in terms of her school achievements and adult accomplishments. Baby B will also be happier and more emotionally stable.

This book, then, deals with the first three years of your child's life. A quick look at the chapter headings will give you an idea of how we have chosen to present the material. The first four chapters cover the first year of life in three-month increments: birth to three months, three to six months, six to nine months, and nine to twelve months. The next two chapters are devoted to the second year of life: twelve to eighteen months of age and eighteen to twenty-four months of age. The final chapter covers the two- to three-year-old period. I have chosen to break down the chapters in this manner because of the speed of the child's growth and development. During the first year of life, new milestones are reached almost on a daily basis and as she gets older the rate of growth and development slows down.

Each chapter will be quite specific in its recommendations and suggestions. Appropriate tables showing growth and developmental milestones will be included in each chapter. It is my hope that this format will make it easier for you to achieve the goal of all parents – to allow your child to achieve the very best possible that is in her, intellectually, emotionally, and physically.

The growth and development charts found in each chapter refer to the expected normal milestones of full-term babies (thirty-eight weeks gestation). If your baby is born prematurely, you must factor this in while checking the charts. For example, a baby born at thirty-four weeks gestation will be one month behind in his growth and development. It often takes up to two years for a premature baby to completely catch up. As long as she doesn't fall further behind month by month with her developmental milestones, there is no reason to worry. There are also normal ranges of development that must be taken into account. If you suspect that your baby is not growing or developing at a normal rate, it is important to discuss this with her doctor as soon as possible. As is the case with just about everything, the earlier a problem is identified, the better the chances of fixing it. My frame of reference in presenting this material is somewhat different from that of the child psychologist who deals almost exclusively with psychological and emotional development. As a pediatrician I must deal with the whole child, and this also includes her physical well-being. By physical well-being I do not mean only the prevention of disease. Rather, I espouse the concept of physical vigor and well-being based on proper exercise, nutrition, and the prevention of obesity. We will be dealing with these aspects of your child's physical development in each and every chapter. We will also discuss safety tips and injury prevention, chapter by chapter, in relation to your child's age, and we will try to explode many of the myths and old wives' tales associated with child rearing. For example, allowing a nine-month-old who enjoys standing and jumping up and down to do so will not cause her to grow up bowlegged. On the contrary, it is good exercise and will help her develop agility and strength as she happily bounces around.

Before going any further, I would like to establish some ground rules. First of all, the concept of normal ranges of growth and development must be clearly understood. Just as in the case of reading a thermometer, when temperatures of 98.6° F. or 99.4° F. are considered within the normal range, there are normal ranges of developmental milestones. An infant who sits without support at seven months of age is just as normal as a six-month-old who does the same. You must always keep this in mind, both when reading the growth and development charts and when reading the text. It is a fact that many parents are overly concerned with how soon their babies start to talk. There are tremendous normal variations in language development from child to child. Some babies start to talk before their first birthday and others don't utter a word until they are two years old. The early talker is not necessarily the more intelligent child. The important thing to look for is how rapidly the child learns to understand words and phrases. Only when a child falls outside the normal range of growth and development should a parent become concerned and consult the doctor. Each and every child (including an identical twin) is unique and each one grows and develops at her own individual rate. This concept is so important that it will be repeated and emphasized over and over again throughout the book.

This book was not written to make it easier for you to compare your child with your neighbor's child, nor, for that matter, to compare her with an older brother or sister. Comparing one to another is not only a waste of time, but may actually be destructive. Further, it has not been my intent in writing this book to make it easier for you to set unrealistic goals for your child. You may very well want your three-year-old to grow up to be a neurosurgeon or another Derek Jeter, but my best advice is to keep those expectations to yourself. Nor is my purpose to motivate you to spend every waking moment figuring out ways to push and pressure your child into becoming the "best" in everything. Overburdening you baby will actually slow down her development.

I have not written this book to substitute for or infringe upon your baby's doctor. It is extremely important that you find the proper physician for your child, either a pediatrician or a family physician who takes care of infants and children. Aside from the doctor's experience, credentials, and hospital appointments, he or she must be available when needed. No matter how good his or her training, if the doctor you have selected or his or her substitute is never around, it is unacceptable. Emergencies do arise and they must be met. If you find that you never can communicate with the doctor, especially during times of emergency, you would be wise to think about making a change.

The so-called "well-baby" visits usually scheduled every two months during your baby's first year, and less frequently after that, are misnamed. Too many parents believe that the only reason for these periodic checkups is to allow the doctor to administer the various "shots" (immunizations) needed. While it is true that immunizations are essential for optimal health, this is not the main reason for these examinations. Only through these regular office visits can your baby's doctor assess your child's growth and development and pick up any slight deviation from the normal early enough so that effective treatment can be given. These examinations also allow the doctor to diagnose an illness that you may not be able to recognize. Your doctor will also check your baby's vision and hearing. Among the major causes of poor academic achievement are impaired vision and impaired hearing. If a defect is picked up early enough, it can be corrected more easily. And, important for your own feelings of confidence and security, during these sessions you will have the opportunity to ask your doctor questions and discuss any problems that have arisen since the last visit.

Many well-meaning parents practice "crisis medicine." This means that the only time the infant or child is taken to the physician is when she is ill. This is absolutely wrong and can lead to irreparable and irreversible damage. By keeping up the so-called "well-baby" and "well-child" visits to your doctor, you will give your child a much better opportunity to develop optimally in all areas.

Finally, I have not written this book to help instill guilt. There is no question that many parents are anxious and unsure of themselves. It is my hope that reading the information in my book will allay much of this fear and insecurity. All that parents can be expected to give is the very best they have in them. It would be unrealistic and foolish of me to expect anybody to follow to the very last detail each and every suggestion and guideline presented. Let me assure you that there are many successful methods of raising children. I am simply offering my approach for your consideration. I believe that following many of my recommendations will make it easier for you to be a positive parent. If you find that some of what I write is impossible for you to follow, or if you disagree with any of my suggestions, or if your baby's doctor has different ideas, so be it.

Authorities in child development agree that parents do not have to be well-educated or enormously intelligent to give their child the best possible start in life. There is really no reason to feel inadequate or upset if you do not have a Ph.D. from Harvard. As a matter of fact, some of the best and most successful parents I have ever known have had a minimum of formal education.

It is not easy to be a parent today. As we enter the twenty-first century, new census data demonstrate that for the first time fewer than one-quarter of all households in the United States are made up of married couples with children. The number of families headed by women grew nearly five times faster in the 1990s than the number of married couples with children, and this trend has continued in the 2000s. Well over half of mothers with school-age children and half of mothers with preschool-age children are now working outside the home. Further, one out of two marriages ends in divorce.

There are some who believe that the concept of "family," however it is constructed, has become outdated and obsolete. This group argues that the only real and important entity is the individual. I don't agree. As far as I am concerned, the family still remains the most important unit in our society. The interrelationships, or "family life," that tie the various members of a family together are the vital core of our society. I believe that these family interrelationships between parents and children are critical to the optimum development of the child. Various social and economic pressures put an enormous strain on the family. Both mothers and fathers are forced to spend many hours away from their homes and their children. It is therefore even more important that the time spent with the child be "quality" time.

This gradual erosion of our family structure is wreaking havoc with many of our children, and the trend must be reversed. I cannot emphasize strongly enough that there is nothing more important than the "family." Bringing up your own child and taking pride and satisfaction in doing the best job possible is what it's all about. The obligation to be a real parent to your child should be, but unfortunately often is not, the most powerful drive in today's society. The prime responsibility of parents is to work together to raise their children properly and to help build strong family ties. Character is built; nobody is born jealous or selfish. Parents should learn to use the word "our" rather than "my." Although it should be obvious, many parents do not realize that children learn by example. Even small infants are attuned and responsive to what goes on around them. I will never forget talking to the parents of a two-year-old boy whose entire vocabulary at the time consisted of "shud up" and "shid." By the time he was three he could properly pronounce his t's.

During the first few years it is particularly important that a close, nonrejecting, stimulating, trusting, and responsive relationship be established between parents and child. If this close and enduring relationship is not developed, lasting detrimental effects on the future emotional and intellectual growth of the child may result. Many studies have clearly shown that early exposure to factors that stimulate a child's interest and motivate her to higher and higher achievement influence and affect her level of functioning when she starts school. Parents should do everything possible to encourage their children to share their ideas and accomplishments with them. This kind of environment is a most important ingredient in the development of intelligence. A baby's intellectual development is closely tied to her feelings. The two really cannot be separated. Therefore, in order to develop to the fullest intellectually, the child not only needs activities and stimulation, but also the confidence to know that she can do it (self-esteem). She must also believe that these activities are worth doing. This requires you to show not only love but also pride in her accomplishments, while at the same time not expecting too much too soon. You can never encourage your child too often or too much and you never should stop showing her and telling her how proud you are of her achievements. Building up sufficient self-esteem and self-worth early on in your child's life is probably the most important way to nurture and guarantee her future emotional health and well-being. If this is successfully instilled, your child will be well on her way to a happy, fulfilling life. A truly loving parent should share her child's discoveries and enjoyments. Be very careful not to put down you child, but rather praise her for her accomplishments. Remind your child at every opportunity how much you love her, how proud you are of her, and how happy you are to have her.

The right attitude and intentions give you a good start. But it takes more than that to be a truly positive parent. It takes a detailed understanding of your child's growth and development. It requires separating fact from fiction. It requires specific knowledge, whether it be about nutrition, safety, toys, games, activities, bonding, trust, or self-esteem – step by step, age by age. Learning what to expect and when to expect it and what you can do to help as your child rapidly grows from infancy to three years of age, ready and well-equipped to face school and the outside world, is what I hope you will gain from this book.

You are competent for the task. There is nothing complicated, magical, or mystical about child rearing. Parents need specific guidelines and direction, depending on the particular age of the child. This book is my attempt to help you reach your goal of giving your child the very best possible start in order to achieve her maximum physical, intellectual, and emotional growth and potential. You will never have a more satisfying and important challenge.

Birth to Three Months

The big day has finally arrived. After nine months of waiting, your baby is born. This is a hectic period for all concerned. The proper equipment and supplies must be on hand in order to satisfy the physical needs of the new baby. Drastic changes in sleep schedules and workloads for both mother and father are the order of the day. Sleeping late on a Sunday morning and reading leisurely through the newspaper are things of the past. It isn't easy to allocate time properly so that everything gets done. This is all obvious, and there really is no reason to dwell on this aspect in any great detail. What it all comes down to is the establishment of proper priorities.

If you are a fastidious, compulsive homemaker, you will simply have to let your housework go if it interferes with your spending enough time relating to and interacting with your new baby. It is easier and more satisfactory for all if both the mother and father share the various new chores right from the start. If this happens, the "family" will be starting off in the right direction. There is nothing unmanly about a father changing his baby's diaper or giving him a bath. I have been pleased to observe that in recent years more and more new young fathers are participating more fully in actively caring for their new infants. Nonetheless, there are still too many new mothers who are over-ly possessive of their newborns and always talk about "my" baby. This type of mother makes it more difficult for the father to share in the rais-ing of their new baby, even if he really is anxious to do so. I would like to remind you that all of us are born with forty-six chromosomes, twen-ty-three of which come from the mother and an equal number from the father. All things being equal, a new baby is entitled to the loving care of both mother and father. Such a baby has a distinct advantage over the baby who has only his mother to care for his needs. If we can all agree that fathers are equally important and responsible for child care, perhaps we can bring about changes in the workplace and public policies that would allow both parents time for parenting as well as work.

SLEEP

Sad to say, your new addition will "not sleep like a baby" through the night. He will sleep many hours each day (average is 16½ hours per day 24 hours) but will wake up frequently during the day and night. Some babies sleep as little as 10 hours per day and some sleep as much as 22 hours per 24 hours, all perfectly normal at this age. This is similar to adult sleep requirements. Some of us require 9 hours sleep per night and oth-ers only 5 hours. To help your infant sleep, soft music or the simple sound of a fan sometimes works. I would suggest that you allow your baby to become accustomed to the usual noise level in your house, rather than trying to keep everything too quiet. However, while your baby is asleep I would not encourage you to practice if you are a drummer by profession.

I have been upset through the years by the fact that many new par-ents do not realize just how important these first three months are for their baby's emotional and intellectual development. The emphasis of child rearing during this period is usually placed almost exclusively on the physical needs of the infant – feeding, changing, cleaning, bathing, and the like. Of course these areas are important, but the new infant has many other needs that are just as important. Many parents are completely unaware of the fact that the first three months of an infant's life comprise a period of not only rapid physical growth but rapid intellectual and emotional growth as well.

Strong evidence indicates that infants from very early in life have many adaptive capabilities. A baby is not a lump of clay to be molded and shaped by his parents; each baby has a complex personality and each is unique in his potential. A baby starts developing from the first moment he is born. An infant's developmental powers come from within. These powers obviously are helped by the environment surrounding him. Not only is the infant influenced by his environment, but he in turn influences the environment as well. The earlier that parents realize this, the better. During the first three months of life, infants frequently smile before they are smiled at, look at people before they are look at, and, of course, communicate by crying. The result is that an infant attracts the attention of the people around him. By their own efforts infants often increase the degree of stimulation of their environment. This is a difficult concept for many parents to accept, but if you do, it will help you tremendously in your child-rearing activities. As the mother of a two-month-old girl recently told me, "You know, Dr. Eden, Amanda is a real person and very nice. She's fun to have around." I wish more new parents would feel this way.

If you are the one out of the thirty mothers who gives birth to twins, the most important thing to remember is that each of your babies, even if they are identical, is a separate, different, and distinct human being. Each grows and develops at his own pace, and so they should never be compared to each other. The incidence of twin births has increased in recent years, due mainly to the more frequent use of fertility drugs. In 1980, before these drugs were readily, available the incidence of twins was about one in sixty, according to the 2005 National Vital Statistics Report from the Center for Disease Control and Prevention.

The reality of being a parent of twins is that you will have twice as much work. Some good advice is to try to take care of both twins together. For example, if possible, feed and bathe them at the same time. In some cases they can be breast-fed together, one on each breast. Alternate the position of the twins with each feeding, so that you don't play favorites. Keeping track may be difficult. Mrs. G. solved that problem by designating her twin girls A & B and her breasts A & B. She established alternate schedules, an A & A and B & B feeding, followed by an A & B and B & A feeding. I didn't believe her but she insisted that her system worked. If your breast milk supply is not adequate for both babies or if it is too difficult to breast-feed both at the same time, breast-feed one and formula feed the other, again alternating with each feeding. Most mothers of twins find the that this combination feeding method works best. Accept all the help you can get.

Twin parenting can be very tiring. When you find that it all just seems too much for you to handle, just think about the poor mother who has triplets.

The simplest way to look at it is that during this period almost all your baby's needs can be taken care of right in your arms. His main physical need is proper nutrition, and a baby should be held while being fed. His emotional needs can also mainly be satisfied by holding, and a good part of his intellectual stimulation is achieved by playing with him as you hold him in your arms. New babies respond to warmth and cuddling. Security and comfort are conveyed through the feel of the mother's or father's body. Love is conveyed through touch, so don't skimp with the holding and hugging. Love is also conveyed by verbal contact – tone of voice, a point many parents do not realize. A newborn hears clearly right from the start.

A normal infant makes rapid and dramatic progress in growth and development physically, emotionally, and intellectually during the first three months. In the growth and development charts that follow, I have listed some of the important developmental milestones that your baby will achieve. As I have already stated, there are normal ranges, and each and every baby progresses at a different rate. These charts are simply guidelines so that any large deviation can be called to the attention of your baby's doctor. One point to remember is that these charts (and the charts in subsequent chapters) refer to full-term infants. A premature baby often will grow and develop at a slower rate and may take two years or longer to catch up with the full-term infant.

The growth and development charts are divided into three sections:
1. Physical (motor)
2. Emotional (social)
3. Mental or intellectual
Turn the page to find the growth and development charts.

GROWTH AND DEVELOPMENT

PHYSICAL (MOTOR)

BIRTH - 1 MONTH

- Thrusts out arms and legs.
- In sitting position, head falls backward or forward.
- On stomach, can lift head slightly and briefly.
- Usually holds hands in fistlike position.
- Rolls slightly to side while on back.

1-2 MONTHS

- On stomach, lifts and holds head up.
- Brings hands together in front.
- On back, turns head to side.
- Makes voluntary movements of arms and legs.
- When held in sitting position, holds head fairly steady.
- Begins voluntary grasping.
- May hold object for a few seconds.
- May start to swipe at nearby objects.

2-3 MONTHS

- On stomach, can lift both head and chest up.
- Usually hold hands open.
- Able to sit supported with head held fairly steady.
- Actively moves arms and legs, usually both arms and both legs together.
- Starts to reach for nearby objects, usually without success.
- May grasp a rattle placed in fingers.
- Turns head efficiently from one side to another.
- When held steady, starts to support part of weight on legs to stand.

Note: These charts are based on average ranges of growth and development; many normal babies perform and achieve either sooner or later than indicated.

GROWTH AND DEVELOPMENT

EMOTIONAL (SOCIAL)

BIRTH - 1 MONTH

- Pays attention to sounds, especially familiar voices.
- Stares at faces and objects with vacant expression.
- Starts eye-to-eye contact.
- Usually stops crying when held and cuddled.
- Cries for help and when in pain.

1-2 MONTHS

- Smiles when you smile or play with him.
- Smiles on his own; starts showing happiness.
- Squeals and makes throaty and cooing sounds.
- Enjoys bath and being held, handled, and played with.
- Listens attentively to various sounds.
- Quiets down when held or in response to familiar voice or face.
- Can quiet self by sucking breast, bottle, or pacifier.

2-3 MONTHS

- Smiles easily and spontaneously.
- Laughs, squeals, chuckles, gurgles, and coos.
- Alertly turns head toward speaking or singing voices or other sounds.
- Recognizes mother or other primary care person.
- Starts to try to attract the attention of anybody around.
- Need for social stimulation more and more apparent, e.g., when talked to, responds with various sounds.
- Begins to distinguish different speech sounds from other sounds.
- Feels upset and protests when left alone.

Note: These charts are based on average ranges of growth and development; many normal babies perform and achieve either sooner or later than indicated.

GROWTH AND DEVELOPMENT

MENTAL (INTELLECTUAL)

BIRTH - 1 MONTH

- Can focus eyes poorly.
- Vague, vacant expression on face while awake.
- Quiets being held.
- Can fix gaze on light or large nearby object.
- Cries for help.

1-2 MONTHS

- Can focus eyes more efficiently.
- Stares at surroundings, preferring person to object.
- Can follow light or moving object to midline.
- Becomes animated and excited when anticipating activity, such as feeding.
- Associates a particular person with a particular activity, e.g., mother and feeding.
- Studies own hand movements.

2-3 MONTHS

- Begins to demonstrate memory.
- Starts to recognize and differentiate various family members.
- Follows with his eyes from one side of his head all the way around to the other.
- Can look at one object or person and then at another.
- Explores his own mouth, face, and other body parts with his hands.
- Can turn head and neck efficiently to look for source of sound.
- Becomes bored and irritated when not sufficiently stimulated with activities.

Note: These charts are based on average ranges of growth and development; many normal babies perform and achieve either sooner or later than indicated.

There is often an overlap between social and mental milestones and they really cannot be separated in any meaningful way. Therefore, the same activity may be listed twice. Since advances are so rapid during the first year of life, the charts of this chapter and the following three chapters are broken down into one-month increments. These charts are incomplete in the sense that they do not attempt to list everything your baby will be doing each month. However, they do list what I consider many of the most important milestones. Becoming familiar with what to expect and when to expect it will make the specific suggestions and recommendations that follow more meaningful and easier to carry out.

With the growth and development charts in mind, I'd like to go on to the specific recommendations that will get your infant off to the best possible start physically, emotionally, and mentally.

PHYSICAL (MOTOR) DEVELOPMENT
NUTRITION

Proper nutrition is most important in helping your baby reach optimal physical health and well-being during these first three months. Unfortunately, many of our current infant-feeding practices are faulty, often leading to obesity, iron-deficiency anemia, and increased strain on the kidneys. The possible long-term implications of inadequate and faulty nutrition may include coronary heart disease, high blood pressure, adult obesity, and loss of I.Q. points.

The ideal way to feed an infant during the first three months and beyond is to breast-feed. Human milk has been shown to be ideally suited to the infant's nutritional needs. Furthermore, there is strong evidence that in addition to being nutritionally excellent, breast milk contains antibodies that protect your baby against certain viral and bacterial infections, especially those involving the gastrointestinal tract. Results of large-scale investigations support the theory that breast-fed babies may be better able to handle cholesterol in later life than those who were bottle fed. Breast-feeding also reduces the number of middle ear infections. Studies have shown that breast-fed infants are protected against certain types of cancer. Of particular importance are the results of a number of studies demonstrating increased intelligence in breast-fed babies. One example of this comes from a recent Swedish study demonstrating that infants who were breast-fed from at least three months had a higher average I.Q. score at five years of age then those who were not breast-fed or were breast-fed for fewer than three months. Another study from the National Institute of Child Health and Human Development compared the cognitive development of 299 children who were born with normal weight and 220 children born small for gestational age. In both groups, the babies who were breast fed for at least three months averaged a 4-5 I.Q. point increase, as compared to infants who were not breast-fed or were breast-fed for fewer than three months. On top of all that, breast-feeding is easy, hygienic, and economical. Further, breast-feeding is also beneficial to the mother. It helps prevent osteoporosis and hip fractures later in life, allows the mother to get back in shape more quickly, and also protects against breast cancer. I am pleased to tell you that, in fact, more and more mothers today are choosing to breast-feed, as compared to twenty or thirty years ago. But we still have too many women who decide not to breast-feed. I believe that the message about the tremendous advantages of breast-feeding, both for the baby and the mother, has not been heard by enough people. Many health care workers just don't take the time to educate mothers-to-be about the importance of breast-feeding or have not themselves been taught enough about this subject. We recently conducted a survey of all the OB/GYN and pediatric residency training programs in the United States to determine the level and quality of the breast-feeding education residents received during their training. Many program directors in both disciplines believed that both the level and quality of breast-feeding education were either fair or poor. What is also disturbing is that too many mothers who leave the hospital stop breast-feeding too soon. Fully one-half of mothers who start breast-feeding stop by three months. One of the main reasons for this is more and more mothers now work outside the home and believe that once they go back to work, breast-feeding must stop. Wrong! The supply of breast milk is determined by how often the baby is put on the breast for feeding. If suckled less often, the milk supply decreases. Therefore, there is absolutely no reason to stop breast-feeding after going back to work. Your baby will happily drink from a bottle (either stored breast milk or formula) while you are away and will breast-feed without a problem when you are home.

If at all possible, I strongly recommend that you breast-feed your baby for at least the first three months of life. The longer you continue to breast-feed, the better. There are very few valid medical reasons not to breast-feed. It is the best way to satisfy all the emotional and nutritional needs of your baby. Many mothers make the mistake of not thinking enough about whether or not they want to breast-feed during the pregnancy. This is the sensible time to decide. But too often the decision is made only after the baby is born. As a pediatrician, there are times when I do not see an infant until he is brought into my office at two weeks of age drinking formula. Obviously, it is then too late to discuss the many advantages of breast-feeding. When I do have the opportunity to talk to the mother during her pregnancy or examining the newborn in the hospital, I do my best to encourage breast-feeding. What I am about to write may not sit well with some of my obstetrical colleagues, but I believe that as a group, obstetricians are not as knowledgeable or interested as they should be in presenting the case for breast-feeding during the pregnancy, explaining the many advantages, both for the mother and for the baby. Of course, the ultimate decision must rest with the mother, but how can she make a sensible choice of breast-feeding versus bottle feeding if she is not aware of the huge advantages of breast-feeding?

MYTH: Breast-feeding will damage the contour of the breasts and cause them to sag.

There is absolutely no evidence that this happens. If a mother maintains her proper weight and does the appropriate exercises, breast-feeding will not change the shape of her breasts in any way. Time and gravity are what causes sagging breasts.

When breast-feeding is unsuccessful, inappropriate because of lifestyle, stopped before three months of age, or simply if the choice is made to bottle-feed, there is no reason to feel guilty about it. Although I always encourage mothers to breast-feed, I disagree with those in the pro-breast-feeding community who take the position that it is a crime not to do so. This overzealous group has not yet come right out and advocated prison for such a mother, but they sometimes come close. The commercially available iron-fortified formulas provide the most rational and desirable alternative to breast milk for meeting all the infant's nutritional needs. Although not identical, they are quite similar to breast milk in their nutrient mix. In addition to being very close to breast milk in the amount of carbohydrates, fat, and protein they contain, commercial formulas also have comparable concentrations of minerals and vitamins. There is no question that from the nutritional point of view, babies do very well on these formulas.

A few words about cow's milk allergy. If your baby is drinking formula and develops gastrointestinal symptoms such as diarrhea, vomiting, bloating, or blood in the stool, he may be suffering from a cow's milk allergy and his doctor should be consulted (infant formulas are made from cow's milk). If the symptoms are due to a true cow's milk allergy, the formula should be changed to a non-cow's milk–based formula. The allergy is due to the protein in the milk and not due to lactose intolerance. Although lactose intolerance is common in adults, especially among Blacks and Hispanics, it is very rarely seen during the first three years of life. Your child's doctor will decide what type of formula to use.

For the bottle-fed infant, the Committee on Nutrition of the American Academy of Pediatrics recommends that an iron-fortified formula be used for the first year of life to prevent iron-deficiency anemia. There is no reason to ever use a formula that is not iron-fortified. The whole subject of iron-deficiency will be discussed more fully later on, since this seldom is a problem during the first three months of a baby's life.

MYTH: Iron-fortified formula causes constipation.

No! This is simply not true. The iron in the formula just makes the stool a little darker.

Whether you breast-feed or bottle-feed, an important point to remember is not to overfeed your baby. How can an infant be overfed? One way is by not allowing your baby to decide when the feeding is over. I find this happening more often among bottle-feeding mothers than among the breast-feeding group. The reason is that the bottle-feeding mother knows exactly how many ounces of formula she starts with, and come hell or high water she will see to it that every last drop gets down the baby's throat. The breast-feeding mother has no way of knowing exactly how many ounces her infant consumed, and so the feeding stops when the baby is satisfied and satiated and stops sucking vigorously.

Remember that it takes at least three hours for an infant's stomach to empty after an adequate feeding. Therefore, if your baby is crying one or two hours after a feeding, it is unlikely that he is crying from hunger. Many new parents automatically assume that every time a baby cries he is hungry. This just is not so. Infants cry for many other reasons. They cry when they are lonely, thirsty for water, gassy, or cranky, and sometimes they cry for no apparent reason. The fact that an infant will drink some of the bottle or suck on the breast does not necessarily mean that he was really hungry. Sucking is a normal reflex in all infants. Overfeeding is an inappropriate feeding practice. In the long run it can lead to obesity, and along with obesity comes inactivity. This all results in less than optimal physical health.

It is relatively easy for you to recognize if and when your infant is being overfed. During the first three months of life a baby should gain on average about one and a half pounds per month. If he is gaining well over two pounds each month he may be overfed. An infant who is bottle-fed and gaining weight too rapidly can be slowed down by giving him formula diluted with water. For example, if your baby is taking six ounces per feeding, each bottle can be made up with four ounces of formula and two ounces of water. Before diluting the formula you should, of course, consult with your baby's physician. If he agrees that your baby is gaining weight too fast he may advise you to cut down on caloric intake. It is more difficult to do something about excessive weight gain in an infant who is breast-fed. We still have not figured out a way to dilute breast milk. However, studies show that many breast-fed babies who have gained excess weight during the first few months of life slim down more rapidly later on than bottle-fed babies with the same degree of obesity.

It has been my experience that the incidence of obesity later on in life among bottle-fed babies is greater than among the breast-fed group. Recent large-scale studies have shown this to be true. I believe that this can best be explained by the fact that the average breast-feeding mother is less frantic and tense and tends to overfeed less often. Further, breast-feeding mothers often begin giving their infants solid foods later than bottle-feeding mothers.

MYTH: Solid food helps a baby sleep through the night.

Despite what you may have heard to the contrary, there is no real evidence that this is true. All authorities on infant nutrition agree that for the first three months, solid food is not only unnecessary for desired growth and development, but actually is contraindicated. The too-early introduction of cereals, fruits, and the like supplies the infant with unnecessary extra calories and also may cause colic and other gastrointestinal problems. There is even some evidence that this too-early introduction of solids predisposes a child to food allergies and asthma later on in life. In my own practice, I start infants on solid foods between four and six months of age, and in the next chapter I will give you my specific suggestions and schedules. It is difficult to convince some parents and it is especially difficult to convince grandparents that solid foods should be withheld during the first three months. Nevertheless, your infant will be better off if you go along with this recommendation. This reminds me of an interesting telephone conversation I had with a new mother who called me up at five o'clock one morning asking me if she could start her eight-day-old baby girl on some cereal. I confess that I was not quite as pleasant as I usually am in answering her. What I said (for which I apologized later on) was the following: "No, you certainly can't start the baby on cereal. However, I certainly would recommend pizza with sausages and anchovies."

For these first three months of life, your baby should be kept on a diet consisting exclusively of breast milk or a commercially available iron-fortified formula. Unless there is a specific reason for the supplemental iron or vitamins, as for example for a premature baby, milk or formula is all your baby needs. Water may be given between feedings, starting at two months of age for breast-fed babies.

Let me take care of two other common misconceptions:

MYTH: Air conditioning is harmful for my baby.

Wrong. Your baby's temperature is no different from your own. If the temperature in your house is such that you are more comfortable in an air-conditioned room, the same holds true for your infant. Nowadays most hospital nurseries are air-conditioned, so there is no reason for you to worry about air-conditioning. Your baby will be much more comfortable and content in a cool (not cold) environment rather than in a hot, stuffy room. A temperature setting between 68° F. and 70° F. is ideal.

MYTH: Flashbulbs should not be used to take pictures of little infants.

Wrong again. There is no reason not to use flashbulbs since they do not damage your infant's eyes. Go right ahead and snap away. I hope your photographs turn out sharp and clear!

EXERCISE

Aside from proper feeding practices, you can do a good deal more to help your new baby develop strength, agility, and muscle tone. Remember that acquiring motor skills helps intellectual growth as well. Your new baby is not a fragile object to be handled with care because he may break. On the contrary, new babies are quite sturdy and well-engineered. There is no reason to be afraid of handling or moving them around. Your main precaution should be to support your infant's head for the first month or so, when it is quite wobbly. Infants are most often carried around in the so-called burping position up on your shoulder. I would suggest that you carry him around in different positions as well. This helps strengthen his large muscles. An infant seat or a pack-sack can be used for this purpose. The baby can sometimes be positioned face forward and sometimes face backward. Not only will this help his physical development, but it is more interesting for the infant as well. Strengthening the infant's neck muscles and helping him achieve good head control should also be part of his activity schedule. The way to do this is to place him on his stomach a number of times each day while he is awake. This will give him the opportunity to learn to lift his head off the surface. There is no question that babies love to be handled, bounced up and down, and exercised. The earlier you start, the stronger and more agile your baby will get. There is an additional exercise that is useful. When the infant is lying on his back, his legs can be exercised by pumping them gently as if he is riding a bicycle. You will find that along with his enjoyment of the activity, all the muscles in his lower extremities will be strengthened.

Various crib devices are useful in stimulating physical activity. They need not be elaborate, and you can make them yourself. If you do, be certain that they are sturdy and solid. There are a number of different crib devices that can be purchased. One example is a cradle gym. These devices, with rings and bells attached, are hung over the crib. A baby will start to swipe and reach at around two to three months of age, and this gives him an excellent opportunity to exercise. Incidentally, he also will be very pleased with the noises he produces when he actually hits his crib device.

Optimal physical development requires more than just feeding, bathing, and changing the infant. It requires exercising and handling and moving the baby around. A flabby, inactive infant is not as healthy as a toned-up active one. The future physical well-being of your infant begins right now.

Safety is a major factor in caring for our children. Thus, in this chapter and in all subsequent chapters, I will list a number of important safety tips immediately after the section dealing with the physical aspects of your child's development. I am sure you would agree that a serious accident such as a severe burn or the ingestion of a poison will adversely affect and tragically, sometimes permanently, interfere with optimal health and well-being.

SAFETY TIPS

Sleep position. It is very important to put your baby to sleep on his back, never on his stomach. This protects him from the tragedy of sudden infant death syndrome (SIDS). There are no exceptions to this rule. Since the Back to Sleep campaign was started in 1994, when parents were taught about this, the number of babies dying from SIDS each year has decreased dramatically. In October 2005, the American Academy of Pediatrics recommended that a pacifier be used at bed-time and at nap time, starting at birth for formula-fed babies and at one month of age for breast-fed babies (to ensure that nursing is well-established) to further reduce the chances of SIDS. This recommendation was based on the body of research that supported a protective effect of pacifiers against SIDS.

Co-sleeping (Bed-sharing). In 2005, the American Academy of Pediatrics Task Force on SIDS also recommended that infants not bed-share during sleep. However, if you choose to sleep in the same bed as your baby, it is important to avoid soft sleep surfaces, for example, sleeping together on a couch. Blankets, especially bulky ones, pillows, comforters, or other soft materials should never be placed under or around the baby. The risk of SIDS has been shown to increase if you smoke and co-sleep. It is well-known that drugs and alcohol can impair your arousal from sleep.

Therefore, if you bed-share with your baby, you must not smoke, drink exclusive, or take drugs, which of course is also good advice if you don't co-sleep. Finally, be careful of headboards or railings, since a baby can get his head trapped between the mattress and the railings or headboard.

Never smoke when carrying your baby. Your may wonder why I have included this tip, as it seems so obvious. Please believe me when I tell you that through the years I have had to treat many small infants who have been severely burned by a cigarette. While we are on the subject of smoking, I would like to make a general plea to all parents to stop smoking. This would not only be best for the health of your small baby, but also for your own welfare. A number of studies, both in the United Sates and Scandinavia, have proved conclusively that during the first year of a child's life he is particularly vulnerable to respiratory infections. It has been shown that the infant living in a house with smokers has a much greater chance of being hospitalized before his first birthday because of a severe respiratory infection than the baby who lives a smoke-free environment. Tobacco smoke exposure also increases the risk of developing asthma later in life. Perhaps this knowledge will motivate you to give up cigarettes. I would also advise you to cut out cigarettes during pregnancy, since it is clear that smoking can damage the developing fetus.

Never leave your baby unattended while he is on any surface from which he can fall. Recently I hospitalized a two-and-a-half-month-old who suddenly decided to turn over for the very first time. Unfortunately, this happened while he was on a dressing table when his mother went to answer the telephone. The result was that he fell off the table, landed on his head, and suffered a cerebral concussion. Happily, he recovered without any permanent damage.

Never hold your infant while riding in an automobile. This method of automobile traveling is unsafe. An infant seat specifically designed for automobile travel should always be used, and it should be one in which the baby faces backward. The trip home from the hospital nursery should be the first time your infant uses an appropriate automobile infant seat. Unfortunately, I do not see this happening often enough and the result has been many infant injuries that could have been prevented.

Never leave your baby alone in a room with a pet, even a lovable, even-tempered dog, and never leave him alone with any child under six years of age. Obviously, I am also including any other uncaged pet – a cat, hamster, guinea pig, bird, etc (teddy bears don't count).

Never shake your baby vigorously, since it can result in severe brain damage. I am referring to Shaken Baby Syndrome or Whiplash Syndrome. If an infant is held around the chest and shaken vigorously it can cause intracranial hemorrhage (bleeding in the brain), which can result in brain damage or even death. The shaking causes tears in the blood vessels in the brain. The signs and symptoms may include seizures and respiratory arrest. The usual story is a sleep-deprived, upset parent holding and shaking a screaming colicky baby in frustration. Of course, there are cases of Shaken Baby Syndrome that are obviously due to full-blown anger and deliberate child abuse. The point to remember is that tragically it can also happen to a caring, loving parent who accidentally shakes his or her baby too hard. The important point to remember is never shake your baby, even when happily playing with him.

Never keep your baby in direct sunlight (more about the dangers of the sun and skin cancer later on). Move your baby into the shade or under the stroller's canopy.

Hearing. Although not specifically a safety tip, I want to include danger signals related to hearing difficulties during the first three months of an infant's life, because poor hearing can threaten a child's well being in many ways.

1. Your newborn baby does not startle in response to a sharp clap within three to six feet of him.
2. Your two-month-old does not awaken from a sudden loud noise in his room.
3. Your three-month-old does not blink to loud noises when awake.

If this is the case with your baby, notify your doctor immediately.

Fever. Why include anything about fever with safety tips in this birth to three month chapter? Because fever, even a low-grade fever, is more significant during these first three months than when your child is older. Any rectal temperature above 100.4° F. (38° C.) must be reported to your baby's doctor – it could mean a serious problem.

I would like to briefly discuss immunizations here, immediately following safety tips, because it is unsafe for your baby not to be immunized at the appropriate times, usually starting at two months. I am disturbed that some parents still do not realize how important these immunizations are in protecting against many serious and life-threatening diseases. Parents have been lulled into a false sense of security because widespread immunization programs have reduced the incidence of so many infectious diseases. Some parents are afraid of possible serious side effects from the immunizations. A good example of this was a recent highly publicized scare about the possible association between the measles vaccine and autism. The fact of the matter is that many studies have conclusively proven that there is absolutely no relationship between the measles vaccine and autism. All the vaccines recommended are completely safe.

Despite all the scientific studies proving that the current routinely recommended vaccines are perfectly safe, the whole subject of immunizations remains controversial. The most recent scare about vaccinations was related to thimerosal, a mercury-containing preservative that was found in some vaccines. A great deal of publicity – TV, newspapers, and books – suggested that thimerosal caused autism but in fact there was absolutely no validity to this claim. The adverse publicity did result in the manufacturers voluntarily removing thimersol from all the vaccines that are recommended for infants and toddlers. Of interest is that the prevalence of autism has not decreased since thimerosal was removed, further proving that thimersol was not associated with autism. There are very few valid reasons to postpone any immunization. Even if your baby has a cold with fever, it is perfectly safe to vaccinate at that time. The bottom line – it is your job to make certain that your baby gets immunized on schedule. The entire subject of autism will be discussed in the two- to three-year-old chapter.

It is important to remember that the dangers from many of the diseases immunizations prevent are most serious during the first year, when the infant's central nervous system is most vulnerable. The schedule for immunizations recommended by the American Academy of Pediatrics must be followed, and the primary series should be completed by age two.

If you think that I'm using scare tactics, you are right. I have seen too many preventable tragedies through the years because children, for whatever reason, were not immunized and protected on time.

EMOTIONAL (SOCIAL) DEVELOPMENT

The two key words at the core of starting your new baby on the road to optimum emotional development are bonding and trust. The development of bonding and trust describes what your most important job will be during the first three months of your infant's life.

BONDING

What do we mean by bonding? This concept in parenting is of prime importance. A good deal of convincing evidence has accumulated emphasizing the significance of the infant's early emotional and social attachment to and interaction with his mother and father. This bonding process appears to be crucial in determining many future aspects of the child's personality and the relationships he will establish throughout his life with his parents and peers. It has been shown in some excellently designed investigations that as little as sixteen hours of close contact between the mother and infant during the first three days of life can modify the emotional quality of the relationship between them in ways that can be determined and detected as long as one year later.

From the very first time you hold your new baby, you are starting to communicate your feelings, and your newborn gets the message. The emotional bonds that are created between newborn and parent seem to be similar to the process of "imprinting" in animals, the process by which the young of many vertebrate species identify the social milieu to which they belong and to which they will turn for interaction. We know more about animal imprinting then we know about newborn bonding in humans. The critical periods for imprinting have been established in certain animal species. We are uncertain what critical periods exist in man, but it is clear that the first few days and weeks are extremely important. Largely as a result of our knowledge of the importance of bonding, increased attention is being paid to the circumstances surrounding delivery and newborn care in the hospital. Having fathers present during the delivery is becoming more and more accepted. Some hospitals now allow fathers to be present during caesarean sections. Rooming-in arrangements for mothers and their babies are being made in more and more obstetrical hospital units.

Contact between mother and infant immediately after birth is important to the development of positive effective attachments later on. However, infants who miss this earliest bonding experience are not necessarily doomed to a life consisting of poor relationships. There is no reason to be upset if, for whatever reason, you weren't close to your newborn right after delivery. As long as you are aware of the need, you can take steps to compensate later, even if you could not be close to your child immediately after birth.

The most reasonable way to look at bonding is that although it can't begin too early, whenever it starts it is a continuing and ongoing process that never stops. There is strong evidence that the first three months of life are crucial in terms of bonding. The lack of sensory stimulation – holding, touching, taking to, singing to, laughing with the baby – is called emotional deprivation. Without such stimulation and interaction, the deprived infant will find it difficult and sometimes impossible to form positive emotional attachments to other people later on in life. Most authorities agree that social and emotional deprivation cannot be separated from intellectual deprivation.

It has also been found that a mother who does not develop a close and intense attachment to her infant by the end of the third month has already clearly indicated to the child that he is unwanted. This can have devastating effects in the future.

Before leaving this discussion of bonding, I'd like to reemphasize the fact that there is now strong evidence that fathers can bond as effectively and meaningfully as mothers with their newborn infants. Paternal bonding has not been given the attention it deserves. There is nothing magical or unique about mother-infant bonding, though a large segment of the population believes there is. Unfortunately, the role of the father in terms of newborn care has been played down through the years. The stereotype of the father whose main and primary function during the first couple of years is to be the breadwinner of the family, and who leaves the day-to-day child rearing exclusively to his wife, is no longer acceptable. As a matter of fact, effective fatherhood really should begin during the prenatal period, before the baby is born. The degree of a man's concern and involvement with the physical and emotional health of his pregnant spouse and the unborn baby often will be a good predictor of just how effective he will be as a father and is the best way to start the infant on the road to future emotional stability and intellectual accomplishment.

TRUST

As far as the infant's emotional needs during the first three months of life are concerned, the other important key word is trust. It is clear that a feeling of trust should be instilled in your infant starting on day one. It is very important that your baby gets the feeling that the world around him is reliable and that all his needs will be met. A newborn really only has one way to communicate his needs to you and that is by crying. Rather than worrying about your baby's crying, you should consider crying a very useful tool. I would disagree with those who take the position that it is all right to allow an infant to cry without responding in order not to "spoil" him. This attitude certainly will do very little in building up trust between you and your newborn. Babies cry for many reasons: hunger, thirst, gassiness, being wet or soiled, loneliness, overtiredness. Babies have different cries to express different needs and this is their first step in learning to communicate. Your main job is to become attuned to your baby and his needs. In most cases this is not too difficult. It usually takes only a few days or weeks for you to be able to recognize why he is crying so that you can respond appropriately. There will be times when you will not be able to recognize and understand why your infant is crying and it becomes a matter of trial and error for you to solve the problem. Let me assure you that almost every infant is unhappy and irritable some of the time. This is inevitable, so you need not assume any guilt. When you don't know why your baby is crying or fussy and irritable, my best advice is to pick him up and hold him. This approach will not spoil him. Rather, it will start to build up his trust in you, and nothing is more important than that.

Let's get down to specifics.

Respond to your infant's needs. If he is crying, hold him. Newborn infants are relatively helpless and can only communicate their needs to you by crying. No, you won't "spoil" your baby by picking him up when he is crying during these first three months.

Spend time with him. New babies are social, responsive, and need your company. The time you spend with your infant is vital to his emotional and physical development, and you should be happy to want to share this time with him. If at all possible, keep you baby close to you while you are moving around the house.

Communicate with him. Although the new infant does not understand the meaning of your words, he does understand and respond to your tone of voice. Try very hard to speak to him in a soothing, gentle manner and smile and laugh and sing to him.

Hold him – the more the better. The best way you can convey your feelings of love to your infant is through touch. I remember joking with the mother of nine-day-old Joaquin, who was cuddling and singing to him, "I see you like your baby." "He's wonderful." They were getting off to a great start.

Feeding. Breast-feeding is the ideal way to satisfy your baby's emotional needs. The close contact that occurs during breast-feeding does much to establish trust between you, and it is continuing an ongoing bonding process. Bottle-feeding can also be a time for building up trust and bonding. It is most important to hold your baby when you feed him a bottle of formula. There is no excuse for ever propping up a bottle. Every baby needs the security and love that go along with the feeding, which includes holding and touching.

Build up your baby's self-esteem. It is never too early for this. Each and every achievement and accomplishment for your infant should be properly acknowledged. For example, if your baby learns to hit his cradle gym, he will respond with joy to the noise and motion. At such times you should also respond with joy to his achievement and tell him so with a hug and kiss and a smile. Your reaction will reinforce his pride in having learned the skill and will go a long way toward making your baby think well of himself. You may be surprised that I am using terms such as "pride" and "accomplishment" and "self-esteem" in describing what a two- or three-month-old can feel. Don't be. The sooner you realize that your infant's emotional needs are no different from a five-year-old's – and no different from your own, for that matter – the better for both of you.

SOOTHING TECHNIQUES

Some babies are more difficult and fussier than others and just cannot settle down and sleep, even after an adequate feeding. They are not hungry but still stay awake, cranky, crying, and restless. Just as with adults, babies are programmed genetically in terms of their temperaments. Some babies are relaxed and content, others more tense and fussy. Some babies suffer with infantile colic during their first three months, experiencing repeated episodes of screaming for long periods of time, often at the same time each day. If your baby fits into this category, discuss it with his doctor.

The following are a number of soothing techniques that can help your baby quiet down and sleep (Grandma may know some others):

Rhythmic sounds: The hum of a vacuum cleaner or fan or the rhythm of a dishwasher often calms a baby.

Singing: A soft lullaby or nursery rhyme. If it works, keep using the same song. Babies enjoy repetition.

Warm bath: This works for some, but others hate it.

Music: I'm a firm believer in music for people of all ages, including little babies. It's soothing and interesting and makes you feel good. How loud should the music be? If you can't talk over it, it's too loud, which reminds me of a recent wedding we attended.

Massage: Again, some babies enjoy being gently stroked, others can't stand it.

Cuddling: This soothing method gives your baby a secure feeling and as far as I'm concerned, the more the better. Kissing while cuddling is highly permissible.

Walking the floor: Carrying your baby around can become tiring, but think of the calories you're burning up.

Rhythmic rocking: In your arms or in an automatic baby swing is effective.

Pacifier: Some babies can only be quieted down with a pacifier. But its important to use a pacifier for the right reason – which means after an adequate feeding when the baby can't settle down and needs some extra sucking. Pacifiers should not be used as a plug to keep the baby quiet.

Tummy on lap: Place your baby on his stomach, across your lap on a heating pad or hot water bottle. At times, simply rubbing your baby's abdomen helps.

Gassiness: If your baby is crying because of gas, help him expel it with a lubricated rectal thermometer or infant suppository or by using one of the gas-reducing medications (ask your baby's doctor about them).

Automobile ride: A last resort method, when all else fails. Believe it or not, it works. I will never forget five-month-old Patrick who was driving his parents crazy every day at 1 a.m. Rain or shine he would start screaming uncontrollably, loud enough to wake up all the neighbors. We tried everything but nothing worked. At 1:30 a.m., I got the phone call and suggested to Patrick's father (home alone with his son) that he go to the all-night pharmacy for a mild sedative that I would phone in. You guessed it. They never got to the drugstore. Patrick fell asleep as soon as the car started. There are now devices on the market that simulate the crib going sixty miles an hour that are said to work. I have not had experience with them.

MENTAL (INTELLECTUAL) DEVELOPMENT

It would be safe to say that many parents believe that not much can be done to stimulate and help a baby develop his mental processes during the first three months of life. Nothing could be farther from the truth. As I already explained, a new baby is not just a blob of protoplasm whose only requirements are to be fed, changed, and bathed. One look at the growth and development charts brings this point home. New babies can hear, see, and very early on, react to their surroundings. The key to helping to develop your infant's intellectual capacities during these first three months is to do everything possible to encourage curiosity.

VISUAL SKILLS

You can help your baby develop his visual skills in a number of simple ways. Well-lighted rooms are helpful.

Place your baby in the prone position (on his stomach) a number of times each day. In this position he will be able to raise his head and look around to see more of what is happening around him. If the baby is kept on his back most or all of the time, he will only be able to see what is above him, and in a short time he will become bored and irritable. Even a one-month-old baby thrives on action and activity. Therefore, changing your baby's position and placing him on his stomach makes it easier for him to become involved with his surroundings and other family members.

Put your baby in an infant seat (always remembering to prop him up to support his wobbly head). This upright position allows him to look around the room and follow you with his eyes as you go about your daily activities. During his waking hours your infant will not only be happier but will be more stimulated if he is kept near you rather than allowed to remain in the crib.

During the first three months all infants spend a great deal of each day in the crib. Therefore, it is important to give your baby interesting things to look at while he's in his crib. Little babies become bored, just like you and me (although I hope that you are not bored reading this). It is a good idea to put brightly colored pictures on the walls around the crib. Shiny, bright fabric or foil can be hung from the sides of the crib for the first few weeks of life. After that it would be wise to get rid of them, since by then most infants can start to reach. Mobiles can be hung above the crib, but they should always be far enough away so that the baby cannot reach them. Remember that everything a baby grabs goes straight into his mouth.

HEARING

From the day he is born a baby hears and absorbs every sound around him; you should always keep this in mind. First and foremost, the tone of your voice should always be soothing and gentle. You will be pleasantly surprised at how responsive your infant will be to cheerful voices and sounds around him. Even the youngest infant seems to enjoy music of every kind, the more the better. I remember suggesting to a new mother that she sing to her baby. She became upset and I could not understand why. It turned out that her husband made fun of her singing, which she described as being flat and out of tune. It took awhile for me to assure her that her one-month-old was no music critic, and to go right ahead and sing to her heart's content.

To develop your infant's hearing capabilities, you might also attach bells to his booties. As he kicks, the jingling will please and interest him. This also helps encourage kicking exercises. Always make certain that the bells are securely attached.

OTHER SUGGESTIONS

Crib devices. These devices, which were discussed in the physical-development section of this chapter, are very helpful in stimulating curiosity as well as encouraging physical activity.

Rattles. These really are of only limited value for most infants during the first three months. The infant has trouble holding the rattle and will usually drop it quickly and be unable to pick it up. Some infants are more dexterous than others and enjoy holding and shaking a rattle. The important thing to remember is to make sure that any rattles you buy are large and sturdy and nonflammable. Use brightly colored rattles, since babies can already start to recognize colors.

Repetition. Babies learn through repetition. Memory is developed through repetitive activities. There is a real question as to the exact age when actual memory begins. Most authorities believe that the start of memory begins at around two-and-a-half to three months of age. It is important and useful for you to give your baby the opportunity to repeat various actions over and over again. The repetition process should be looked upon as a real learning experience, one that helps your infant develop his intellectual capacities. An example of learning by repetition would be the use of a hanging crib device with bells attached. The baby sees the device and hits or swipes at it. When he makes contact, the device moves and the bells ring, and when he misses it, nothing happens. As the infant becomes more skillful and dexterous, he succeeds more and more often in hitting the device, and his reward for the achievement is seeing the device move and hearing the sound of the ringing bells. It is never too early to provide positive reinforcement for achievement. When he succeeds, hug, cheer, and applaud and tell him "good job." This is how you start to build up his self-esteem and self-confidence and his desire to learn, achieve, and excel. The more you talk and sing to your baby, the better.

The mother of three-month-old Amy once asked me if I thought it was a good idea if she sang to her in French. "Of course it is," I told her, as long as she sang in proper Parisian French. Incidentally, Amy is now four years old and speaks both English and French fluently.

During the first three months an infant must be allowed to have his natural curiosity satisfied. With the few simple devices and activities I have just described, you will help your new baby achieve his maximum mental growth.

2

Three to Six Months

What can you expect during this period? For one thing, there will be lots of action. Your baby will make some remarkable advances, physically, emotionally, and mentally. Central to these advances will be her ability to learn to deal with things manually. This skill is called prehension, the ability to grasp. Between three and six months of age your infant will begin to grasp for what she sees, tastes, or feels. This skill will allow the baby to gradually begin to learn to bring together the spatial information she obtains. The result of the mastering of prehension is that she will be able to coordinate and relate certain movements to the environment. This manual dexterity is crucial for her normal development.

Your baby will also begin to develop and master hand-eye coordination. She will now be able to reach for the objects she can clearly see. Further, babies begin to roll over, and some begin to creep. It therefore allows the baby to start to explore the world around her.

Let me assure you that during these next three months it will be much easier for you to enjoy your baby and have fun with her than it was during the first three months. Although she will be awake much more than she was during the first three months of life, she will usually be quite cheerful and happy. It is true that teething may interfere with her usual genial disposition, but aside from the discomfort often associated with the teething process, your baby will be very easy to live with.

Recently the mother of a five-month-old girl described her baby as being a "real ham." What she meant was that Yvonne spent most of her waking time performing for her parents in order to attract their attention. Yvonne imitated, babbled, and made all sorts of noises to gain the attention of anybody around her. When her audience responded, Yvonne squealed, chuckled, and kicked her legs in a state of complete euphoria. This description is classic. These three- to six-month-olds really have a happy time of it. They are usually in a pretty good mood even when left alone with their toys. But they almost burst with joy and happiness when the people around them pay attention and respond to their actions. A comedian performing in from of an audience soon becomes discouraged when nobody laughs at the jokes. Your baby is no different. She too will become discouraged and withdrawn if, despite her best efforts, she is not able to get the appropriate response. Her self-esteem gets a big boost when her actions are appreciated and not ignored.

I would like to re-emphasize just how important it is for you to really relate to your baby in every way possible. Although there is not much you can do at this age to speed up development, what you don't do may slow development. Lack of sufficient touching, holding, and talking during these first few months of life results in smaller brains.

The question about a mother going back to work often comes up when the baby is around three months old. This is an important subject and will be discussed fully in the next chapter (Six to Nine Months). You have my permission to skip ahead if you are facing that decision now.

Needless to say, especially for economic reasons, there often is no choice. If that is the situation in your house, there is no reason to feel guilty about it.

A few words about trust and curiosity: Memory and understanding are developing and your baby is becoming more responsive each day. She depends entirely on you to satisfy all her needs, and if you let her down too often, the trust that must be built up between you will suffer. As your baby grows and develops, she becomes more alert and more curious to explore and learn about her surroundings. After the growth and development charts that follow, I will give you specific recommendations to help you help your baby make the most out of these next three months.

On the next page you will find the growth and development charts to help you monitor your child's skills. Remember, these are averages only and many babies perform and achieve either sooner or later than indicated.

GROWTH AND DEVELOPMENT

PHYSICAL (MOTOR)

3-4 MONTHS

- May roll from stomach to back.
- Can sit with propping and support.
- Reaches with hands more efficiently and purposefully.
- Swipes at nearby objects, usually successfully.
- While sitting, holds head fairly steady.
- While on back, can lift head up.

4-5 MONTHS

- On back, lifts up head and shoulders.
- Rolls from stomach to back.
- Sits with head and back steady with support.
- May be pulled up to standing position.
- May hold bottle with both hands or with one.
- Begins to transfer objects from one hand to the other.
- Starts to reach for and grasp objects.

5-6 MONTHS

- On back, can grab feet.
- Can roll from back to stomach.
- Sits without much support.
- Holds bottle well.
- Begins to reach and swipe with one arm at a time.
- Starts to learn to manipulate objects in her hands.
- May grasp small objects off a flat surface.
- On stomach, starts to creep forward or backward with legs and steer with arms.

Note: These charts are based on average ranges of growth and development; many normal babies perform and achieve either sooner or later than indicated.

GROWTH AND DEVELOPMENT

EMOTIONAL (SOCIAL)

3-4 MONTHS

- Smiles at people easily and openly.
- Recognizes mother and father.
- Turns toward familiar voices.
- Enjoys games and socialization.
- Laughs loudly, squeals, and chuckles.
- May coo or sound one syllable, e.g., ooh, ah.
- May smile at mirror image.

4-5 MONTHS

- Recognizes various members of the family.
- Resists when toy is taken away.
- Smiles and makes sounds to gain attention.
- Starts to have angry and fearful reactions.
- More responsive to human voices; turns to look at speaker.
- May start to imitate.
- Plays with rattles, toys, bottles, etc.

5-6 MONTHS

- Can imitate facial expressions and voice inflections.
- Responds to her name.
- Smiles at mirror image.
- Plays games with pleasure and enjoys sound effects, e.g., peek-a-boo.
- Enjoys other children; smiles and touches them.
- Makes "raspberry" sound with tongue between her lips.
- Disturbed and frightened by strangers.
- Responds to music with cooing.

Note: These charts are based on average ranges of growth and development; many normal babies perform and achieve either sooner or later than indicated.

GROWTH AND DEVELOPMENT

MENTAL (INTELLECTUAL)

3-4 MONTHS

- Alert and responsive to surroundings and people around her.
- Reaches for toys that are out of reach.
- Memory span increasing to up to ten seconds.
- Recognizes various members of her family.
- Aware of her hands, and carries objects to her mouth.

4-5 MONTHS

- Awake and alert for longer periods of time.
- Looks down for falling objects.
- Imitates sounds and movements.
- Fearful of strangers and new situations.
- Recognizes familiar objects and people, and reacts appropriately.
- May say vowel sounds and some consonants: b, d, m.
- Memory span continues to increase.

5-6 MONTHS

- Starts to reach for dropped toys.
- May begin to compare two objects at a time.
- Uses her fingers and mouth to explore objects around her.
- Can lift a cup by its handle.
- Can reach for and grasp the things she sees.
- Stares and studies objects carefully and for long periods of time.
- Says many consonants and vowels.

Note: These charts are based on average ranges of growth and development; many normal babies perform and achieve either sooner or later than indicated.

PHYSICAL (MOTOR) DEVELOPMENT

NUTRITION

The main source of nourishment for your baby between three and six months of age should continue to be breast milk or a commercially prepared iron-fortified formula. As stated in the previous chapter, there is universal agreement among pediatricians that breast-feeding is the ideal way to feed a baby. If you have chosen to breast-feed I would encourage you to continue to do so during these next three months. As a matter of fact, the longer you breast-feed, the better off your baby will be. It is recommended that supplemental iron be given to breast-fed infants starting at four months of age, since there is not enough iron in breast milk to prevent iron deficiency beyond four months. Supplemental vitamin D is also recommended at this age. In our office, we put all breast-feeding infants on a multi-vitamin containing iron at four months of age. Discuss this with your baby's doctor. If, for whatever reason, you decide to discontinue breast-feeding any time during these three months, it is most important that you switch to an iron, fortified formula and not to cow's milk. As noted earlier, commercial formulas are specifically designed to meet all the nutritional needs of the infant and so are very close to breast milk in their nutrient mix. Cow's milk may be ideal for baby cows, but it never was designed for human babies. More and more evidence has accumulated pointing to the potential dangers of feeding cow's milk to infants during the first year of life.

If your baby has been fed formula during her first three months, my advice is to continue. There is no need to give supplemental iron or vitamin D, as is the case for breast-fed infants. I am often asked about the total quantity of formula an infant requires during each twenty-four-hour period. I can't give you a direct answer to the question because of infants' variable energy requirements. What I can say is that if you allow your infant to stop each feeding at the first sign of satiation or willingness to stop, it is highly unlikely that she will ever be over- or underfed. As a general rule, after three months of age, very few infants consume more than two-and-a-half ounces per pound per day. For example, a baby weighing twelve pounds will probably not drink more than a total of thirty ounces of formula each day. If your infant has a voracious appetite and is gaining weight too rapidly by drinking tremendous amounts of formula, the simplest way to slow down the monthly weight gain is to dilute the formula with some water. Before doing so, I suggest that you consult with your baby's physician.

What about the introduction of solid foods? A number of surveys have shown that most infants in the United States today are fed some solid food before three months. My experience confirms these findings. All the authorities in the field agree that this is too early for solid foods. The two main reasons for the too-early introduction of "beikost" (meaning foods other than milk or formula) are the belief that they will help the baby sleep through the night (a myth dispelled in the previous chapter) and outside social pressures. Too many mothers seem to compete with each other to see who can feed solids to her baby earlier. I am very upset when I hear parents brag about all the solid food they push down their infant's throat long before the baby requires any at all. We have already stated some of the reasons for not starting solids too early; namely, unnecessary extra calories and the potential for developing allergies later on. Another important reason for not rushing to give your infant solid foods is that doing so can interfere with the establishment of proper eating habits. Since it is important that an infant be encouraged to stop eating when satisfied, she must be able to communicate this feeling to the person who is feeding her. At four to five months of age, most infants can sit with support and have relatively good control of their heads and necks. These babies are able to lean forward and open their mouths when interested in the food, and are also able to lean backward and turn away when not interested or satiated. If solid foods are introduced before the age of four months, the infant will find it difficult to make her feelings known, and this will result in forced feedings. The American Academy of Pediatrics recommends that solid foods be started between four and six months of age and I agree. The key to proper feeding is to allow your baby to decide when the feeding is over, and not to stop the feeding when you think she's had enough. This simple concept will do much to establish correct feeding habits – and these habits will continue as the child grows and develops. They will go a long way to ensure your child a full, active, and healthy future. There is no need to start any solid food at this age. Breast milk and iron-fortified formula meet all the nutritional needs of your baby. Don't stuff her with so much solid food as to interfere with her milk intake.

It usually takes a few days' practice for your infant to learn to swallow from a spoon. I would suggest that you start with just one teaspoon of solid food the first day and gradually increase the quantity each day. It would be prudent to start only one new food at a time and give each for a few days to be sure that the baby can tolerate what she is fed. The signs of food intolerance or allergy are vomiting, gassiness, rashes, and excessive crankiness. If any of these signs develop, simply stop that particular food and go on to another.

The sequence I follow for the introduction of solids varies from baby to baby. Infant cereals are started first. They are all fortified with iron, by law in the United States, and are well-tolerated and seldom allergenic.

Age	Type of solid food	Time
3 months	None	
4 months	Pre-cooked cereals 2 times a day	Morning and evening
5 months	Add strained single fruits 2 times a day	Morning and evening
6 months	Add strained vegetables	Lunch

Your baby's doctor is in the best position to decide when to start and what foods to give. The following is the average schedule of solid foods recommended to my patients for the three-to-six-months period.

Alternate green and yellow vegetables. If you use only yellow vegetables, your baby may develop carotonemia, with resulting yellow skin. This condition is not dangerous but it should be avoided. Cereals are mixed with formula. Fruits and vegetables are fed without adding formula. Always feed with a spoon. It is not a good idea to add any solid food to the bottle.

This is a good time to discuss sugar and salt. It is unhealthy for a baby (and for anybody, for that matter) to eat too much salt or sugar. Whether you make your own baby foods with a blender or use commercial products, do not add sugar or salt. The baby food manufacturers have removed added salt from all their products and added sugar from most, so what remains is the natural-occurring salt and sugar. This was an important forward step in fostering proper nutrition. You should not allow your baby to become accustomed to foods that are either too salty or too sweet. Food tastes and preferences are established early in life. No baby is born a "sugar freak" or a salt craver. Food contains enough natural salt and sugar to take care of all your baby's nutritional needs. Eliminating extra salt and sugar from your baby's diet can help prevent the later development of high blood pressure, dental decay, and obesity.

EXERCISE

Your three- to six-month-old baby loves to exercise. My best advice is to give her the space and allow her to do as much exercising as possible. You do not need to buy any fancy equipment for this purpose. The following are my recommendations for exercising a three- to six-month-old baby:

Crib devices. These have already been described in Chapter 1. Your baby can start to grasp and reach and is becoming increasingly proficient at these activities. She will make excellent use of the device attached to her crib, and this is a good form of physical activity.

Don't swaddle your baby by wrapping her tightly in clothing and blankets. I am totally opposed to this practice. Your baby should be given the freedom to move her arms and kick her legs freely, without restraint. This advice holds true as she gets older as well.

Turn-over games. Babies never seem to get tired of or bored with turning over again and again and gain. This activity is great fun for the baby and is an excellent exercise as well. It does much to tone up the muscles and increase her agility. Although you may get tired of watching her, your baby won't tire of doing it, so give her every opportunity to practice – and react appropriately when she succeeds.

Kicking toys. You can either buy or make your own large cuddly kicking toy and attach it to the sides of the crib. These kicking toys can be a continuing source of pleasure for your baby as she kicks at and grabs for them. These not only keep her busy and happy but also allow her to develop strength in her legs.

Creeping and rocking along. Many five- to six-month-old babies start to creep or push themselves along, either forward or backward. It therefore makes good sense to take your baby out of the crib a number of times each day. Either put the baby on the floor (clear of small and sharp objects) or in a playpen so that she can have the space to practice and develop these new skills. Starting to get from one place to another in order to explore her environment is an exciting time for your baby and you should encourage this form of exercise as much as possible.

Standing. Between three and six months of age, most babies can support their weight while standing supported. Get your baby up on her feet. This will help her develop strength in her lower extremities as well as improve her large-muscle coordination.

As I noted earlier, standing a baby too early will not cause bowlegs. There is absolutely no truth to this old wives' tale. I am often asked by parents about how long to stand a baby up. My answer is, just as long as the baby is happy doing it.

The important thing to remember is that exercise habits start early in life. The infant who is kept swaddled and restricted, is not permitted to begin to explore her environment, and discouraged from exercising every step of the way will very soon become discouraged and inactive. If your goal is optimal physical development, you should encourage your baby to use all her muscles. At this age it is not difficult to give her all the exercising she wants and needs.

SAFETY TIPS

Let me point out that many of these safety tips will be repeated in subsequent chapters. As a rule I don't like to repeat myself, but when it comes to safety I make an exception.

Automobile. Your baby should always ride in a car seat that folds backward in the back seat.

Never leave your baby alone on any elevated surface. Three- to six-month-olds can turn over, and some can creep and move around, so you are really looking for trouble if you leave them unattended. A sensible idea is to use a safety strap.

Smothering. Plastic bags, long toy telephone cords, harnesses, and soft pillows can smother or strangle a baby. Obviously, all these should always be kept away from your baby. A firm crib mattress and loose covering for the sleeping baby are safest.

Small and sharp objects. It is important to keep pills, buttons, pins, beads, and any other small or sharp objects away from you baby's reach. At this age everything goes into the mouth. I will never forget making a house call and finding the five-month-old sick baby lying on her dressing table, securely strapped down. As I started to examine her mouth, I was horrified to see an open safety pin already halfway down her throat. Fortunately, I was able to grab it and pull it out before it disappeared from view. I am not sure who was more upset about this incident, the mother or me.

Burns: Always check the bathwater temperature first to prevent scalding your baby. Never drink hot liquids such as coffee or tea while holding your baby on your lap.

Pets. As previously written, never leave your baby alone with your dog or cat. Pets can be wonderful companions, but they can bite and scratch. They also may harbor worms that can cause disease in humans. Therefore, deworm your pets on schedule, as recommended by the veterinarian, and make sure your pet is properly vaccinated.

Immunizations. As pointed out in previous chapter, it is essential that your baby receive all her immunizations and be fully immunized by age two. It makes no sense at all for so many children in the United States not to be getting all their vaccines on time. In many developing countries, there is not enough vaccine to go around, but in the developed world, there is no such excuse for delaying those routine safe and effective vaccines.

Hearing: The following may be danger signals pointing to hearing difficulties during this period. If you notice either one, tell you infant's doctor about it.

1. Your four-month-old does not turn to the source of a distant sound.

2. Your six-month-old gradually stops her babbling noises.

Sleep: Continue to put your baby to sleep on her back, using a pacifier at bed-time and at nap-time. Your baby's sleep cycle remains short. The result is that she tends to sleep lightly or wakes frequently during the night. This often sets the stage for behavior problems later on. She will now sleep a total of 14-16 hours a day, with many short naps. To help her sleep, keep the temperature in her room comfortable. Many parents overdress their babies and keep their room too hot. A proper temperature to shoot for is 70° F.

EMOTIONAL (SOCIAL) DEVELOPMENT

We are back to bonding and trust. During this period in your infant's life it becomes much easier for you to relate in a positive way. Since three- to six-month-old babies are so alert, cheerful, and responsive, you should find each day interesting, different, and a real adventure. The bonding process that started the moment your baby was born continues. For the emotional well-being of your baby, this positive nurturing relationship between the baby and her parents must be reinforced and solidified every single day.

The actual number of hours you spend with your baby is not as important as how you spend each hour. In discussing this with parents I often use the term "quality time." Just being around and not relating or responding to all your baby's needs is not what quality or positive parenting is all about. I also do not mean just responding when your baby cries. When she is cooing or gurgling or laughing, she also is communicating her feeling to you, and you should respond in kind. Show affection by holding, kissing, cuddling, and talking to her in a soothing, loving voice. Your little baby understands exactly what you are trying to get across to her. All your baby needs is your love, so why skimp on it or ration it out?

Parents often ask me if there is any way they can determine if they are, in fact, giving their baby enough love and affection. Since there is no way to measure these, there is no real answer to their question. All I can say is that mothers and fathers who are thinking about this aspect of parenting are on the right track and most probably are satisfying their baby's emotional needs.

MYTH: A baby who is frightened by strangers is insecure and unloved!

Absolutely not. Somewhere between four and six months of age, some babies develop a fear of strangers. This can be considered normal behavior. The fear disappears in time and is nothing to worry about. This reminds me of a recent experience in my practice. Baby Elizabeth, age five months, was upsetting her parents enough to bring her to my office to find out if there was anything wrong. It seems that Elizabeth, a happy, healthy, and friendly baby, screamed with fright every time Grandma came to visit and picked her up. It took me quite awhile to convince the family, including Grandma, who also came along, that Elizabeth was perfect in every way, and that there was no reason to be concerned. Incidentally, by the time Elizabeth was nine months old her favorite visitor was Grandma.

During this period your infant wants very much to keep everybody around her amused. She turns and kicks and reaches, and she laughs and giggles and coos. She deserves to have her performance appreciated, especially by the people closest to her. I once got a 10 p.m. phone call from the mother of a five-and-a-half-month-old baby. She was bursting with pride and happiness as she told me what had just happened. While changing the baby's diaper, Mrs. T. suddenly sneezed. Baby Emily gave out a big belly laugh in response to the sneeze, and both mother and baby then had a mutual laughing session. Momma actually could not wait to share this happy experience with her pediatrician. I was quite happy hearing the story, but I was even happier that Mrs. T. hadn't sneezed at 3 a.m.!

GAMES

There are some simple games that you can play with a three- to six-month-old, games that your infant not only will enjoy but that will also increase the bonding and trust that are so essential for a baby's emotional well-being.

Peek-a-boo games. Make them up as you go along; they all work fine.

Tickling games. Baby loves to be tickled at this age and giggle and laugh in response.

Drop-the-spoon game. Usually by five to six months of age infants learn to reach for dropped objects. They also enjoy having you pick up the spoon and can't wait to drop it again. This is great fun for them, but sometimes not such great fun for your aching back.

This little piggy went to market. Wiggle each of her toes as you say the lines.

Making faces. Infants at this stage are learning to imitate and have a marvelous time doing so.

Many parents do not realize how important it is for them to regularly play with their babies. I have mentioned previously and will continue to repeat that feeding, changing, and bathing are not enough. Your baby deserves more out of life than that, and it is so very easy for you to give it to her. Sharing fun games together is a must.

Infants are very attuned to their surroundings. Emotional stability is nurtured by friendly, familiar, affectionate voices, laughter, and singing. Babies also require and respond to close physical contact. There is no such thing as too much touching, holding, and carrying around.

MYTH: A baby is spoiled by "too much attention."
In my opinion, just the opposite is true.

MENTAL (INTELLECTUAL) DEVELOPMENT

Sometimes between three and six months of age your baby will begin to show signs of intelligence as we usually understand it. The question as to the actual age intelligence develops is a favorite of infant-developmental psychologists. I would say that intelligence begins on the day of birth. Nevertheless, the usual signs that we associate with intelligence become obvious between three and six months of age. The infant now learns to use her hand as a reaching tool under the guidance and direction of her eyes. Your little baby will now simultaneously see, reach, and touch. Besides this establishment of efficient hand-eye coordination, your baby will now show real interest in the objects she can reach, and so it makes good sense to give her as many interesting objects as possible to look at, feel, and handle.

SPECIFIC RECOMMENDATIONS

The following are some specific recommendations for stimulating your infant to develop her intellectual capacities to the fullest between three and six months of age.

Use an infant seat. Move the location of the infant seat frequently to change your baby's environment. Try to keep her near you in her infant seat as you go about doing your chores. Keeping her close to you rather than isolated in another room not only will result in her being happy and pleased to have your company, but will also open up many opportunities for learning.

Take your baby outside. Frequent walks in the carriage will do both you and your baby a lot of good. This will encourage and stimulate her interest in the outside world. The more she sees and the more she is exposed to, the better.

MYTH: Babies catch cold if taken outdoors during cold weather.
Colds are caused by a number of different viruses, and babies catch cold from being exposed to another person who is carrying a particular cold virus. These upper-respiratory infections have nothing to do with the temperature outside. As a matter of fact, it has been my experience that infants who are taken out into the fresh air are healthier as a group than the ones who are cooped up inside most of the time.

Talk to your baby. You may think it strange that I suggest talking to your baby, since it is so obvious. Let me assure you that many parents simply do not realize how crucial it is for them to talk to their infants at this age. They wrongly assume that since the baby cannot understand the actual meaning of the words, they should not bother. Although you may find it difficult at first, try to talk to her as if she's already all grown up. In other words, don't use "baby talk." Starting early this way will help her speak correctly later on. The beginning of language learning starts during this three-month period. If you talk to your baby about what is taking place around her, development of the language-learning process will be stimulated. Many studies have demonstrated significant differences in intelligence later on in life between those infants who were largely deprived of language interchange and those who were spoken to on a regular basis.

Set up mobiles and mirrors. These should be placed over the crib, but far enough away from the baby that she cannot actually reach out and grab them. They can be quite interesting to the infant and serve as another source of learning. Babies at this age enjoy looking at themselves in the mirror and watching the mobiles move around above them. It gets pretty boring being incarcerated in a crib with nothing much to do or look at.

Using a playpen. There are differences of opinion regarding the usefulness of playpens at this age. I think they are quite useful. While in a playpen your baby is safe, and you do not have to continually watch over her, as you would have if she were allowed to play on the floor. Her playpen should be stocked with interesting, safe objects such as rattles, plastic balls and containers, spoons, and lids of pots. Banging pots and pans seems to be one activity that almost all babies enjoy. Clutch balls and squeaky toys also should be provided. Supplying your infant with a variety of these objects allows her to play by herself for long periods of time without becoming bored. They also give her the opportunity to learn more rapidly. These same objects can also be used while your baby is in her crib.

Imitation. This is an important mental skill that usually starts around five months of age. The infant begins to imitate various signs and movements, and this should be encouraged by you. The first step in imitation learning is for you to copy the things the baby does. In short order she will begin to understand what you are doing and start to do her own imitating.

Sounds and voices. Let your baby hear as many different sounds as possible, such as a clock ticking, the vacuum cleaner, music, the radio, and so on. Give her the opportunity of hearing not only your voice but the sounds you are making as you move about and work in the house. This can only be done if you keep her near you as much as possible.

Your baby is eager to learn and to explore her environment. It is very easy for you to help her attain intellectual development during this period, as you can see by my specific recommendations. You do not need expensive or elaborate equipment, just your time.

3

Six to Nine Months

This period in your baby's life has been aptly called the early exploration stage. By this time he has developed many of the skills that make it possible to interact with and explore the world around him. As the growth and development charts that follow indicate, he will now be able to reach efficiently for and grasp objects, even very tiny ones. Babies at this stage have excellent control of their hands and are fascinated with manipulating the various objects they can grab. In addition, a baby's eyes and ears now function very effectively. He can focus well on objects near and far, and can localize sounds without difficulty. He is able to maintain excellent head control and can freely move his head around in all directions. He will be spending more and more time in the sitting position and so will be able to see much more of what is going on around him. During these three months most babies learn to crawl or drag themselves along the floor, and some learn to stand and "cruise" along the furniture. It therefore becomes possible for these babies to start to travel and investigate what is happening some distance away.

As he becomes more and more proficient in turning, crawling, creeping, kicking, and standing, a six- to nine-month-old is even more involved in physical activity than when he was younger. His interest in games increases day by day. A favorite pastime is dropping objects to see what happens next.

It is amazing how well he is now able to concentrate on a particular activity. By repeating the same task over and over again, he finally learns to master it, and remembers what he has to do. I recall talking to the father of a seven-month-old boy. He could not believe that Johnny never seemed to tire of turning over and over and over again. Furthermore, this little fellow took pride and satisfaction in this accomplishment every single time. It is important to always remember that learning a new skill takes a lot of practice, and an appreciative audience speeds up the process. It is also important to understand that an infant acquires skills one at a time. Trying to learn or do two things at a time just doesn't work for a baby.

This is a period in your baby's life when he becomes even more curious about the world around him. He will want to touch and feel and taste everything he can find and hold. It is important that you encourage him and give him the opportunity to expand his skills and his horizons. A couple of years ago the mother of an extremely active and adventurous eight-month-old bitterly complained to me that she was sure Danny was born "bad." I sat her down in my consultation room and asked her why she felt that way. "Dr. Eden, he is a devil. He gets into trouble all the time just to make my life miserable. He crawls around and puts everything in his mouth. Would you believe that yesterday he actually pulled an electric plug out of the wall and tried to put it in his mouth?" It took me fully thirty minutes to convince her that Danny was not "bad" but rather was an intelligent, healthy, and curious young man and that she should thank God that she had such a fine, brave youngster. I also spent a few minutes gently suggesting some simple safety measures that she had better adopt if she wanted to avoid a serious accident.

Teeth are coming in at this time, and some babies suffer more discomfort than others. Despite the fussiness and crankiness that often accompanies teething, babies during these three months basically are cheerful and content.

They smile, giggle, and laugh a lot, and it doesn't take much to get them into a good mood.

MYTH: Teething causes high fever.

Not true. If your baby has a temperature of over 101° F., it is not due to teething.

Despite the fact that your baby is beginning to move around, he will still be confined most of the time to his crib, playpen, or infant seat. It is interesting that he usually does not seem to mind being a prisoner. This is especially true when he is around six to seven months old. By eight to nine months of age he may not be too happy if he is prevented from moving freely about the room. He then will begin to show signs of frustration when not allowed to initiate various explorations and expeditions.

Memory and understanding develop rapidly, day by day. Ideas are beginning to take shape in his busy, active mind. Verbal understanding is starting. He will learn to understand the meaning of some words such as mama, dada, bye-bye. This receptive language development (understanding) is a much more important and accurate measurement of intelligence than expressive language development (speaking). It will be a happy day indeed when he is able to follow the first instructions you give him such as to wave bye-bye. Most babies achieve this milestone sometime during these fascinating three months.

GROWTH AND DEVELOPMENT

PHYSICAL (MOTOR)

6-7 MONTHS

- Sits well with little support.
- Can grasp with thumb and fingers.
- Creeps and then starts to crawl.
- Rolls over, back to stomach and stomach to back.
- Stands with support.
- Holds and handles spoon and cup.
- Gets himself into sitting position.

7-8 MONTHS

- Sits without support.
- Crawls, forward or backward.
- Stands well with support.
- Pulls himself up to standing position, using furniture to help.
- Once standing, usually cannot get back down.
- Can feed himself crackers.

8-9 MONTHS

- Skillfully picks up small objects, using "pincer" grasp (thumb and forefinger).
- Crawls efficiently even with one hand holding a toy.
- Starts to "cruise" along furniture.
- Can crawl upstairs.
- Manipulates one object in each hand.
- May stand alone for a moment.
- Can pull himself up to a standing position, often in the middle of the night; calls for help to get back down.

Note: These charts are based on average ranges of growth and development; many normal babies perform and achieve either sooner or later than indicated.

GROWTH AND DEVELOPMENT

EMOTIONAL (SOCIAL)

6-7 MONTHS

- Often afraid of strangers.
- Start of sense of humor and teasing behavior.
- Understands different tones of voice and meaning of "no."
- Happy to play with toys.
- Wants to be included in games such as pat-a-cake and in social interaction.

7-8 MONTHS

- Still afraid of strangers.
- Attached to mother or primary caretaker and fears separation.
- Demands and shouts for attention.
- Longer attention span and sustained interest in play.
- Pats at and kisses mirror image.
- Upset when confined.

8-9 MONTHS

- Enjoys being center of attention.
- Eager for approval, and imitates play.
- Pleased with audience response to his exploits.
- Selective in the toys he plays with.
- Loves various games, with dolls and blocks, pat-a-cake, peek-a-boo, etc.
- May start to show signs of selfish behavior, e.g., protects his toys.

Note: These charts are based on average ranges of growth and development; many normal babies perform and achieve either sooner or later than indicated.

GROWTH AND DEVELOPMENT

MENTAL (INTELLECTUAL)

6-7 MONTHS

- Can distinguish distances, near and far.
- Starts to understand the implications and consequences of his actions and behavior.
- May say "mama" and "dada" without attaching meaning to them.
- Imitates the speech sounds he hears.
- Memory improving; responds with excitement to repetitions of event.

7-8 MONTHS

- Can solve problems.
- Starts to understand the meaning of a few words, such as his name, bottle, mama.
- Good memory of recent events.
- Says a few words, still without knowing their meaning, sometimes in two syllables.
- Imitates people and behavior, e.g., waving bye-bye, clapping, and pointing to and following what someone else points to.

8-9 MONTHS

- Follows simple instructions.
- Learns to build two-block tower.
- Understands cause and effect.
- May be able to keep a series of ideas in mind, as memory and thinking processes improve.
- Becomes bored more easily with repetition of same games and activities.
- Understands concept of reward.

Note: These charts are based on average ranges of growth and development; many normal babies perform and achieve either sooner or later than indicated.

PHYSICAL (MOTOR) DEVELOPMENT

NUTRITION

It has been my experience that many mothers who have breast-fed their babies stop by the time the infant is six months of age. But, unless there is a specific reason to stop, I would advise that breast-feeding be continued during this six- to nine-months period.

Recent studies have found that breast-fed children are less likely to become obese than children who were never breast-fed, according to Kathryn Dewey, Professor of Nutrition at the University of California, Davis. An analysis published in 2005 concluded that a child's risk of being overweight dropped by four percent for each month of breast-feeding. Why? Breast-feeding teaches self-regulation of the milk intake by the baby and the feeding stops when the baby is satiated, not when the mother decides that the feeding is over, as is the case with many bottle-feeding mothers. I believe that this probably explains why breast-fed babies are less likely to put on excessive weight later in life. This is another reason why I encourage you to continue breast-feeding for as long as possible.

Throughout human history the weaning age has been well over one year, often somewhere between two and three years. There is certainly no reason to stop breast-feeding when your baby is six months old. This leads me to the problem of the mother who chooses, for whatever reason, to go back to work during this period or even earlier. There is little question that a full-time job creates problems for the breast-feeding mother. One sensible solution is to use a bottle for the one or two feedings the mother is away from home and to continue to breast-feed the remainder of the time. These bottle feedings can be with expressed and stored breast milk if possible (or with an iron-fortified formula).

It is of interest that the breast milk supply is regulated by how often a baby is suckled. The more often the baby is breast-fed, the greater the milk supply. Conversely, if a woman breast-feeds less often, her milk supply diminishes. I have had many breast-feeding mothers go back to full-time jobs away from home and continue to breast-feed successfully. What this all means is that just because a mother goes back to work does not mean that she must stop breast-feeding. As I pointed out earlier, the longer a baby is breast-fed, the healthier and smarter he will be.

Babies who have been fed one of the commercially prepared iron-fortified formulas should remain on the formula and should not be switched to whole cow's milk during this three-month period. My reasons for avoiding cow's milk between six and nine months of age are the same as those previously discussed; namely, there is too much protein and salt in cow's milk for the baby's kidneys to handle. And most important of all, cow's milk contains very little iron as compared to breast milk and iron-fortified formula. Preventing iron deficiency is one of the keys to raising a healthier and smarter child. The whole subject of iron deficiency will be discussed in detail in the chapter Twelve to Eighteen Months.

It is a good idea to limit the total amount of formula per day to less than one quart. If your baby is consuming much more than a quart per day, especially if he is gaining weight too rapidly, a simple solution is to dilute the formula with some water. For example, each eight-ounce bottle can be made up of six ounces of formula mixed with two ounces of water. We haven't yet figured out a way to dilute breast milk.

Skim milk should never be used at this age. Parents have recently become more concerned about childhood obesity and many assume that using skim milk makes sense (as is the case in treating adult obesity). The fact is that there is even more salt in skim milk than in regular cow's milk. Furthermore, many studies have shown that skim milk does not satisfy the energy requirements of infants. It has no place in the diet of any baby during the first year of life.

All babies wake up during the night and some who are bottle-fed have trouble falling back to sleep on their own. In my experience, and the experience of most pediatricians, breast-fed babies as a rule do not go back to sleep on their own but rather fall back to sleep while feeding.

More and more of the total infant diet will now be made up of solid foods. The order in which you introduce various solid foods really makes little difference. But what is important is to continue to feed your baby infant cereal, which, as you will recall, is iron-fortified and important in preventing iron-deficiency. Unfortunately, I see many parents starting their six-to nine-month-old babies on a variety of other cereals that are not specifically prepared for infants. Although many of these may be iron-fortified, a good number have iron in a form that is not readily bioavailable and thus poorly absorbed by the baby. For this reason I would strongly recommend that you continue to feed infant cereal to your baby to help supply him with sufficient iron.

For this six- to nine-month age period, turn the page for my recommendations for additional solid foods.

Age	Type of solid food	Time
6-7 months	Plain yogurt	Snack
	Strained meats	Lunch
7-8 months	Egg	Morning (every other day)
8-9 months	Baby juices (no sugar added)*	Afternoon
*Juices should be limited to no more than six ounces a day, according to the latest recommendations of the American Academy of Pediatrics. Juice should be given as part of a meal or snack, rather than to pacify the baby.		

You will note in the above table that I suggest giving an egg only every other day. There is a good reason for this. Eggs certainly are an excellent food nutritionally, but they are also very rich in cholesterol. As adults we are told that we should not eat more than three or four eggs per week in order to reduce our cholesterol intake. It therefore follows that since eating habits and patterns are established early in life, why not also get the baby accustomed to eating an egg only every other day? In subsequent chapters, I will be discussing the whole question of cholesterol in greater detail.

I have included plain yogurt in the table because I believe that it is an excellent food to introduce early into your baby's diet. Yogurt is a milk product and so should be considered a substitute for some of the breast milk or formula rather than as part of the solid food diet. I consider yogurt good for babies for the following reasons:

1. It is well-tolerated and easily digested.
2. Its consistency makes it easy for the baby to swallow.

3. For adults, yogurt tends to be filling and satisfying, and there is no reason to believe that the same does not hold true for babies.

4. Yogurt is a nutritious, natural product that is high in protein and relatively low in calories.

5. For those babies who cut down on their total daily milk intake, yogurt is an excellent substitute.

6. Acquiring a taste for plain yogurt in infancy will make it more likely that your baby will continue to eat and enjoy it as he grows up.

7. Eating yogurt as a snack food throughout childhood is far healthier and more nutritionally sound than eating so-called "junk" foods, which are less nutritious and too high in refined sugar and calories.

Along with the additional foods I have listed in the table, your baby can now also be started on desserts, teething crackers, and various baby "dinners." These are lumpier in consistency than strained foods and prepare the baby for regular table foods.

At around seven to eight months of age, "finger" foods may be started, such as zwieback, teething biscuits, and pieces of banana. By the time they are nine months old, many babies become adept at handling pieces of cheese or a slice of apple. There is little question that these finger foods do not help to maintain the cleanliness of the room where your baby is eating, but they do give him some necessary practice in using his fingers and also in spoon-feeding himself, which usually starts later. Further, babies at this age like to feel the various foods they eat and they should be given that opportunity.

Fruit juices are now being introduced, so a word of caution about so-called "nursing bottle caries." It has been shown that babies who use the bottle as a pacifier, and suck on the bottle containing juice (or milk, for that matter) while lying down for extended periods of time, destroy their teeth. Because of this, some pediatricians recommend that fruit juice only be fed by cup. I see no reason not to give your juice in a bottle. The important thing to remember is that he should drink it only while in an upright position. If your baby must have a bottle to fall asleep, make sure it contains only water. This approach will not only save your baby's teeth, but will also save you a lot in dental bills.

While on the subject of dental bills, I want to remind you about fluoride. This mineral gives excellent protection against tooth decay. The American Academy of Pediatrics recommends that fluoride supplementation start when a baby is six months of age. When the local water fluoride level contains less than 0.3 parts per million, the daily dose of fluoride should be 0.25 mg. If the local water supply contains over 0.3 part per million of fluoride, no supplement is needed. The daily dose of fluoride remains the same until three years of age. If you do not know the level of fluoride in your local water supply, ask your baby's doctor or your local health department. Well water can be checked for fluoride content through your local health department.

Of course even if your water supply is adequately fluoridated, if your baby doesn't drink tap water, he will require supplemental fluoride. Bottled water usually does not contain fluoride. Fluoride may be given via drops or incorporated into a multi-vitamin preparation.

I have nothing against dentists making a decent living, but I am upset when parents do not take this simple step to protect their children from the unnecessary pain and suffering of tooth destruction due to lack of fluoride.

Before completing this section on nutrition I want to briefly discuss childhood obesity. The facts are very clear. Fat babies have a better chance of ending up fat adults than do normal-weight or thin babies. If you notice that your baby has been gaining weight too rapidly, it is important that you talk this over with his doctor. There are a number of ways of determining if a baby is fat. These include weight charts, body mass index (BMI), and the measurement of skin folds with special calipers. As far as I am concerned, the best method of all is the "eyeball" test. Just look at him. If he looks fat, he is fat. It is pretty hard not to notice the rolls of fat and extra chins. One rule of thumb you might find useful is that normally a baby should double his birth weight by five months of age. For example, a baby with a birth weight of seven pounds should weigh around fourteen pounds by the time he is five months old. Thus, if your six-month-old weighs considerably more than double his original birth weight, be on the alert. You should also be aware of an important factor related to obesity. Obesity runs in families. The statistics are as follows: If both parents are fat, there is an eighty percent chance that their baby will be fat. If both parents are thin, he has only a ten percent chance. The message from this is clear. If you or your spouse is fat, you must be especially careful never to allow your baby to gain weight too rapidly. This brings to mind an interesting case. A couple brought their nine-month-old girl to my office for the first time for a checkup. The baby was tremendously overweight, but surprisingly, both her parents were quite slim. Neither the mother nor the father was aware of or particularly interested in the fact that Amanda was so fat. I also was not overly concerned since she was lucky enough to have two thin parents, so that I thought her chance of remaining fat was relatively small. Asking about her history, I quickly learned that Amanda was adopted and there was no information about the weight of her natural parents! Genetics went out the window and we got busy discussing the dangers of childhood obesity. Amanda's diet was adjusted and her opportunities for exercising were increased. I am happy to report that now, at around three years of age, Amanda is probably thin enough to pass the "eyeball" test of any neutral observer.

ANTIBIOTICS

"Dr. Eden, my nine-month-old baby has signs of a cold and a temperature of 102°. Would you please call in a prescription for an antibiotic?" My answer was a simple but emphatic no. I spent the next five minutes explaining to Mrs. K. that an antibiotic should only be used to treat a specific bacterial infection and it would be inappropriate and maybe even dangerous to start an antibiotic without first examining the baby to find the cause of his fever. I am sorry to say that this type of telephone call is not at all uncommon nowadays, not only in our office, but in physicians' offices all over the country.

Why should we be discussing antibiotics in this six- to nine-month-old chapter? I chose this chapter because it has been my experience that around this age babies are starting to be exposed to more and more people – babysitters, in day care, during trips to the supermarket, etc. The more exposures, the greater the chances of a baby picking up an infection, usually of the respiratory tract. Many of these infections are associated with fever and so I believe that this is as good a time as any to explain both the important role that antibiotics play as well as the dangers of their overuse and indiscriminate use.

Before the age of antibiotics, there was very little that could be done to treat and cure many serious bacterial infections. The results were that children became seriously ill and many died. Epidemics were common in those days. We are now fortunate to have at our disposal many powerful and safe antibiotics that are highly effective and often life-saving. What must always be remembered, however, is that antibiotics do not work against viral infections and the fact of the matter is that almost all the infections your young child catches are caused by a virus. The fever that often is part of these respiratory infections should be treated with a fever-reducing medication such as Tylenol or Advil and not with an antibiotic.

I can almost hear some of you saying, "But even if my baby's illness is caused by a virus, why not put him on an antibiotic just to be on the safe side? It can't do any harm and it may do some good." Wrong on both counts. Let me explain why an antibiotic should never be used when it is not indicated.

The first reason is that each and every time an antibiotic is used, it increases the chances of developing an allergic reaction to it. If this happens, that particular antibiotic cannot be used in the future when it might really be needed. Further, it eliminates from use many other antibiotics in the same class. For example, a child who develops an allergy to penicillin will often also become allergic to amoxicillin, the bubble gum–tasting antibiotic so popular now because of its good taste.

The second reason for not using an antibiotic unless it is really necessary is even more important. Bacteria are not stupid. The overuse of an antibiotic leads to bacterial resistance. This means that a specific strain of bacteria builds up more immunity each time it is exposed to the antibiotic until it finally becomes completely immune to it. We already are dealing with some of these smart drug resistant "super-bugs." The staphlococcus bacterium is a good example of this. Very few antibiotics are now effective against it.

There are some infectious disease specialists who are predicting that if we continue our current indiscriminate use of antibiotics, more and more "super-bugs" resistant to any and all antibiotics will develop, so further down the road we will be back to where we started before we had any antibiotics at all.

So, what's the bottom line? Your baby's doctor should be the only one to decide if an antibiotic is necessary. Remember that a great majority of early childhood illnesses associated with fever are caused by viruses and not by bacteria, and so antibiotics are rarely needed. If your child is put on an antibiotic make sure you give the correct dose for the exact number of days prescribed and then if there is any medication left in the bottle, throw it out.

When I started practicing pediatrics, parents would ask, "Dr. Eden, aren't you going to give my child a shot of penicillin?" Today the question has become, "Dr. Eden, can you prescribe the bubble gum antibiotic?" My answer in most cases has always been the same: "No, I am not. It is not necessary, it won't work, and it can do a lot more harm than good."

I am happy to report that this message is starting to get through. In my office last week, I prescribed an antibiotic to a youngster who had a raging, full-blown, draining ear infection. Her mother asked, "Do you really think Amy needs the antibiotic?"

EXERCISE

The motor growth and development chart should make it obvious that your baby is now really ready for a good deal of physical activity. He is able to sit well, is beginning to stand, can pull himself up to a standing position, crawls and creeps, and may even begin to "cruise" along the furniture. He is now able to turn efficiently, both from front to back and back to front, and can pull himself along the ground on his hands and knees.

In my opinion these six- to nine-month-olds do not require any particular exercise program. It is not necessary to buy any special exercise equipment. All your baby needs is the space to move around; he will do the rest. Since he can now crawl, he will not always be very happy sitting in an infant seat or confined to his playpen. He requires wide open spaces – to crawl, creep, pivot, rock along, and cruise. Since he is full of curiosity, he will want to reach every corner of every room, studying everything in sight and trying to put everything he can grab hold of into his mouth. Very few infants at this age need to be encouraged to move around. All you have to do is give them the freedom and opportunity to do so. The only exception is the baby who is markedly overweight. A very obese baby is often content with merely sitting or lying down, preferably with a bottle of milk or juice or a snack to keep him occupied. A vicious cycle is set up. The fatter the baby, the less active he becomes; and the less active the baby, the fewer calories he burns up, causing him to get or grow fatter. Most of his caloric expenditure seems to be the result of chewing and sucking, and this type of exercise burns up very few calories indeed.

Babies at this age are full of life and fun and very anxious to be physically handled. They love to be swung up in the air, bounced up and down on your knee, and are positively ecstatic when their mother or father gets down on the floor with them for some physical tussling and communal crawling. All these activities promote physical vigor, coordination, and agility, and also help to burn up extra calories. Equally important is the fact that promoting and encouraging physical activity at this early age will make it much more likely that your baby will continue to practice and enjoy vigorous physical pursuits throughout childhood and beyond, helping him stay healthy and happy in his life.

I'd like to call your attention to one common mistake many parents make at around this age: buying a pair of walking shoes just as soon as the baby is able to stand.

MYTH: Shoes make it easier for the baby to walk.

As a matter of fact, just the opposite is true. A baby will learn to walk sooner and better if he is allowed to feel the ground underneath him with his feet unencumbered by shoes. My advice would therefore be not to rush out and get walking shoes until your baby is walking well by himself, without support. Besides improving his walk and strengthening his feet, this will also save you some money. If you are worried about warmth, dress him in some light socks — though I warn you that he may find it fun to remove them.

I am often asked about walkers and if it's a good idea to use one. I advise against a walker. Walkers cause many accidents and they don't help a baby learn to walk. On the contrary, since he can navigate around so well in a walker, he may be less interested and less motivated to practice walking by himself. The American Academy of Pediatrics has recommended that parents do not use mobile infant walkers because of the considerable risk of major injury. Most of the major injuries and deaths are due to head trauma, almost always related to falling down stairs.

SAFETY TIPS

Automobile. Continue to put your baby in a car seat facing backward in the back of the automobile.

Accident-proof your house. If you have not yet done so, this is the time to do all you can to prevent accidents, since your baby is starting to move around. One good example of an important injury-preventing technique is using plastic covers on electric outlets. These are available at your local hardware store.

Toys. All your baby's toys should be unbreakable, too large to swallow, and never have points or sharp edges.

Walker. If your baby does use a walker, make certain that everything that is breakable or potentially dangerous is put away. The use of a walker allows your baby to move great distances very rapidly, so you must be on the alert for injuries.

Burns. It is good idea to put guards in front of open heaters and fireplaces and around radiators. I strongly advise that you use only flame-retardant sleepwear for your baby; read labels and ask questions of store personnel before buying.

Sun safety. After six months of age, sunscreens should always be used when taking your baby outside for any length of time. The sun protection factor (SPF) should be at least fifteen. Apply the sunscreen at least thirty minutes before going outside, even on cloudy days. Apply the sunscreen every two hours while your baby is outside, and reapply the sunscreen after he has been in the water learning to swim. Many parents reserve sunscreen for the beach only. Let me remind you that the sun shines just as brightly in non-beach areas.

Why start protecting a baby's skin so early? Because the evidence is clear that the damage to the skin from the sun's rays is cumulative over the years and too much sun exposure can lead to various forms of skin cancer later on in life.

Kitchen. The kitchen should be considered a high-risk room. Always remember to keep poisons such as bleach and cleaning agents locked away or on a high shelf. Stop using tablecloths. One of the worst burns I have ever had to treat was that of an eight-month-old who was crawling along the floor, reached up, and yanked at the tablecloth. Unfortunately, there was a large pot of freshly brewed coffee on the table at the time. The entire contents of the pot spilled over the baby's face, chest, and abdomen. The result of all this was a two-month hospitalization for severe second-degree burns from which the baby thankfully recovered – but the child is now left with permanent scarring.

Drowning. NEVER LEAVE YOUR BABY ALONE IN THE BATH FOR ANY REASON. It takes only a few seconds for an infant to drown, and the water level of the bath does not have to be more than a few inches for this tragedy to occur.

RETURNING TO WORK

Before starting the section about the emotional or social development of your baby, I believe that this is the appropriate time to discuss in depth the important subject of a mother going back to work, which often comes up when the baby is around six months old or even younger.

First the facts: At last count, more than sixty percent of mothers with children over the age of three are working outside the home. So if you have already gone back to work or will do so during the next year, you have plenty of company. There is little question that the mother's decision to go back to work can be stressful and many mothers feel guilty about it. There are two basic reasons for a mother going back to work, and its sometimes a combination of both:

Economic. A number of opinion polls have shown that this is the main reason mothers go back to work. With the high cost of living today, many families have no choice. Without two paychecks, many families could not survive, let alone save money for their child's future education (medical school is very expensive). A single parent rarely has any choice. At last count, almost one-third of all new babies are born to single-parent homes. And so if your economic situation necessitates going back to work, go right ahead, with a clear conscience and no guilt.

Preference. There are mothers who prefer working outside the house, rather than staying home to care for her baby twenty-four hours a day, seven days a week. Aside from the obvious economic advantage of another paycheck, this group, often women with fulfilling careers are happier and more content working. It makes no sense to me to force or shame these women into remaining at home full-time. A depressed, discontented mother who would rather be out will find it difficult to provide quality care or give enough of herself to satisfy all the needs of her baby. Just being home all the time does not automatically translate into a nurturing, involved parent. If you fit this category, my best advice is to go back to work.

A third reason, the wrong reason, for some mothers returning to the workplace is outside pressures. I have seen mothers who prefer staying home with their baby with no economic problems go back to work due to outside pressures. This is ridiculous. An example of this was a recent conversation I overheard at a cocktail party. A female lawyer and recent mother seemed embarrassed trying to explain to her friend why she chose to stay home with her baby rather than resuming her successful legal career. I almost entered that conversation, but decided to mind my own business. That mother, instead of being embarrassed, should have been proud of her decision to sign on for the most important job of all, the job of being a truly positive parent.

"Dr. Eden, when is the best time for me to go to work?" or "How old should my baby be before I go back to work?" The fact of the matter is that there is no specific best time or best age. I have a friend who went back to work as a full-time pediatrician when each of her two children were two weeks old, and everything turned out fine. She was fortunate to have a terrific full-time nanny she could afford. Another friend had grandma around and so she also got back to work soon after her baby was born. Unfortunately, most families are not that lucky. It usually is difficult and frustrating finding the right person or facility for your baby. My best advice is to stay home to nurture your baby as long as your particular situation allows.

Is it harmful to the baby if his mother goes back to work? This is the $64,000 question. Put another way, are children raised at home by their mothers for the first three years of life better off than children raised in day care settings or by surrogate mothers? My answer is, "It depends" – on the quality of the day care or surrogate mother and the quality of the stay-at-home mother. The question cannot be answered simply yes or no.

In his book *The Growth of a Child,* the noted psychologist Dr. Jerome Kagen poses this question: "Do infants attending a well-run responsible group care center five days a week during the first two years of life display different patterns of psychosocial developments compared with infants with the same family background who are being reared in a typical nuclear family?" The results of his study show that children from intact psychologically supporting families who experience surrogate care during the first two years of life resemble home-reared children from the same social and ethnic groups. No significant differences in psychological and social development were noted between the groups. Quoting Dr. Kagen, "A family has a mysterious power which perhaps is one reason why it has been the basic and most stable unit in this and other societies for so long." To this I say, "Amen." A supportive and nurturing home environment is the key to raising a happy child, whether or not you go back to work.

In my experience, children of working mothers do just as well as children of stay-at-home mothers. The quality of surrogate care as well as the quality of home care determine how well the child will do.

The lack of well-run and well-staffed infant and child care services that are affordable continues to be a real dilemma and a cause of constant stress for many families. Unfortunately nowadays, nurturing, competent grandmothers are few and far between.

So what is the bottom line? The ideal situation for a baby is to be born to a mother who does not need to return to work due to economic reasons and who prefers and looks forward with enthusiasm to staying home with her new baby for the next three years as a full-time mother. If such a full-time mother is happy to provide loving and stimulating care, this is the best possible world for her baby.

For those mothers who must or choose to go back to work, there is absolutely no reason to feel guilty about it. Yes, you must face the fact that working mothers often find combining work and motherhood tiring and stressful. But with the proper support system, be it grandma, daddy, nanny, friend, or a quality child care facility, your baby will do just fine. You will not be able to spend as much time with your baby as you would like, but if the time you do spend is happy, nurturing, quality time, you have nothing to worry about.

EMOTIONAL (SOCIAL) DEVELOPMENT

Your little baby is now full of curiosity while becoming more and more aware of his surroundings. He will start to show signs of humor, demand attention, distinguish different tones of voice, and learn to recognize himself in a mirror. His attention span is lengthening and he is becoming selective in his activities. He continues to enjoy audience response to his exploits and never seems to tire of performing for close friends. He also will develop fear of being separated from his mother and remains frightened of strangers.

SPECIFIC RECOMMENDATIONS

The specific recommendations that follow will help your baby achieve the very best in emotional stability and maturity during this time. They are in large measure the same recommendations I wrote about in the two previous chapters, but they are equally important now. The appropriate games and toys will be covered in the section on mental development, but it is clear that many of the activities specifically geared to help your baby develop intellectually will also help his emotional and social development.

Tone of voice. As I have already stated, this is more important than you may think. Keep your screaming and yelling to a minimum. The axiom you must never forget is that children learn mainly by example. Although your baby may not yet understand the actual meaning of the words you use, he certainly knows the difference between angry words and happy words. It is not easy to maintain a cheerful and loving disposition twenty-four hours a day, especially when you are overworked and tired from lack of sleep, as parent, of young children often are. Nevertheless, you should do your best to be as relaxed and calm as possible while you are with your baby.

Sounds. Babies at this age are very interested in all sorts of sounds, and so it is a good idea to have a radio or record playing as often and for as long as possible. Human voices and music are pleasurable for the baby and give him a sense of well-being and security, especially when you are not around.

Quality time. When you are with your baby, try to give him your undivided attention. I can guess what you are thinking. How in the world can I get all my work done if I have spend so much time playing with my baby? Obviously, there are limits to what you can be expected to do, especially if there are other children in your family or you are working outside the house. However, you should think about priorities. For example, what is more important, a vacuumed rug or a happy baby? The interesting thing about all this is that if you spend "quality" time with your baby, you will build up enough trust and self-esteem in him so that he will be less demanding and clingy. A baby who is encouraged to develop a positive self-image by parents who spend quality time playing and interacting with him is more likely to be happy by himself with his thoughts and toys. During these times you can get the vacuuming done.

Mood changes. Rapid mood changes occur very frequently. Be prepared for them and do not worry about them. The most emotionally stable baby is likely to show these dramatic changes in disposition; they are not signs of emotional deprivation.

Stranger anxiety. The fear of strangers is quite common throughout most of these three months. Your baby is becoming more selective and discriminating and is no longer attracted to each and every person he sees. It would be a mistake to force him to stay with a so-called "stranger" (even if the stranger is your favorite uncle) if he is frightened by it.

Privacy. All of us need some time for ourselves, and your little baby is no exception. If he is playing quietly and happily, practicing his many motor and beginning verbal skills, he should not be distracted. For example, if he wakes up from a nap in a good mood, babbling away and playing with his toys, leave him alone. He will let you know soon enough when he becomes tired of being by himself.

Spanking or yelling. It is an utter waste of your time to try to force your baby to obey you at this age. He can't understand what you have in mind, so spanking or yelling are not only ineffective, they frighten him as well. If he enjoys smashing dishes, for example (which was a favorite pastime of my son at this age), simply remove them from his vicinity and give him something unbreakable to drop instead.

Feelings. Your baby is a little person with feelings that are no different from yours or mine. We all seem to forget this from time to time. Keeping this in mind will make it much easier for you to respond to his needs and get through some of his "bad" days. All of us have days when, as the old saying goes, "It just doesn't pay to get out of bed." The very same thing holds true for your little baby.

Reading aloud. I believe that this is a good time to start reading to your child at bedtime. This ritual should be continued for as long as possible. At this age he will not understand the words or even the simplest story you read, but it will be very useful in promoting closeness, warmth, and comfort before he goes off to sleep.

A final thought before we leave this section: What really counts most is for you to like being with your baby and for your baby to like being with you. If you feel happy together, there really is no way you can go wrong.

MENTAL (INTELLECTUAL) DEVELOPMENT

Between six and nine months of age your baby will make tremendous advances in his intellectual capacities. With a little help from you, he will be able to sharpen his mental skills to satisfy his continuing thirst for knowledge. He will begin to learn the consequences of his behavior, and start to imitate and even understand the meanings of a few words. His memory will get better each day and he will start to solve simple problems.

SPECIFIC SUGGESTIONS

The following are specific suggestions that I believe will assist your baby in achieving his full mental development during these three very interesting months of his life.

Reading. Why discuss reading in this section on mental development? A six- to nine-month-old can't say much, but he is starting to understand what you are saying, so now is the best time to start reading to him. The late Dr. Peter Susczyk, a well-known researcher of infant learning, studied six-month-olds' and proved that they associated meaning with particular sounds or words. They were shown videotapes of their mother and father on different monitors as a voice and said "mommy" or "daddy." The babies looked at the correct monitor often enough to indicate that they understood the association. Reach Out and Read (www.reachoutan-dread.org), a wonderful national organization that distributes books to parents in pediatric clinics and hospitals all over the country based on the age of the child, starts at six months of age and continues to six years. If you start now, your baby will become accustomed to books and reading early on and will become smarter because of it. Reading books to your little baby instead of letting him watch television is the best advice I can give for his intellectual development, and the earlier you start, the better.

Imitation. This can be divided into two separate parts. In the first, imitate his sounds, such as his clapping, banging on a table, or even throwing things. Take the lead from your baby. As he does something, simply imitate his action. This will teach him what imitation is all about.

The next step is for you to make simple sounds to him, such as da, pa, ma, clicking your tongue, or coughing, asking him to imitate you. If he learns to respond, it is the real beginning of word vocalization.

The second part of imitation involves games. Examples would be waving bye-bye, clapping your hands, and an old-time favorite, pat-a-cake. For those of you who may be unfamiliar with this seventeenth-century rhyme, it goes as follows:

Pat-a-cake
Pat-a-cake
Baker's man
Bake me a cake
As fast as you can
Roll it and pat it
And mark it with a B

And put it in the oven
For baby and me

I must admit that before researching this book, I only knew the first five lines, and so my two children were taught a shortened version by their pediatrician-father.

Talking. The idea is to talk to your baby while showing him with gestures what you mean. For example, hold your arms out and say, "come," as you reach to pick him up. Say, "bye-bye," and wave your arm at the same time. When you say, "no-no," to him, shake your finger. This is the time to start teaching your baby the meaning of words. If, for example, he is eating hot food, tell him that it's hot. If he touches hot water, tell him that it is hot. If you do this often enough, he will learn the meaning of the word, and he will not forget it. If you are consistent and do not try to teach him too many meanings too rapidly, he will make steady progress. As I have already pointed out, many mothers and fathers make the mistake – unknowingly, of course – of not talking much to their baby until he starts talking himself. Six- to nine-month-old babies can learn the meaning of some words without being able to say them. Firstborns usually speak earlier than subsequent siblings. The reason is that a parent spends more time talking to the first baby simply because there is more time to do so. With the birth of the next child the workload increases. Now there is less time to talk to the newest baby because his older sibling demands more and more of your attention.

Mirror. A mirror is an effective method for teaching your baby to recognize himself. Put him on your lap facing a mirror and say, "Look, there's Billy" (unless your baby's name happens to be Robert).

Problem solving. This is extremely important in stretching your baby's mental capacities. Figure out ways of giving him something to think about by creating simple problems. For example, place an object in his way as he crawls along. Instead of always handing him his rattle, sometimes hide it behind you or off to one side and shake it to get his attention. He will then learn to localize the sound of the rattle and will take off after it. When he finds it he will be overjoyed, and you should be too.

Play objects. The more, the better. Always make sure that the objects you supply are not small enough for your baby to swallow. Some favorites are balls, stacking toys, plastic cups, soft blocks, and squeaky toys.

Television. Isn't it too early to discuss T.V. in this chapter? No, isn't. As a matter of fact, infants are the fastest-growing T.V. market segment. Researchers reported in 2007 that forty percent of infants are regular viewers of T.V. by this age. A recent large scale study showed that seventeen percent of babies younger than one year were already watching at least one hour per day of T.V. Therefore, this is the age for you to start thinking about T.V. and your baby. Is there any evidence that T.V. watching at this age helps your baby learn, no matter what the content? No, there is not. The American Academy of Pediatrics recommends that children under two years of age should not watch any T.V. at all. I don't completely agree with that recommendation, but I certainly agree that there is no place for T.V. for your six- to nine-month-old baby.

GAMES

Rhythm games. These are lots of fun, besides being an important tool for learning. I am referring to such masterpieces of poetry as this little piggy went
to market; one, two, buckle my shoe; and hickory, dickory, dock. These
and many others are available on records. Another good idea is to play
music and dance and sway to the rhythm or, if you prefer, clap your hands
in time to the rhythm of the music.

Dropping games. These can be a problem for parents with a bad back. As a grandfather, dropping games are now out the question for me. Your baby will
learn to pick up, hold, let go of, and drop an object, and he becomes an
expert in short order. He also never tires of this activity. One sensible
suggestion would be to keep handy a bag full of objects to be dropped
such as spoons and cups. Hand the baby one object at a time from the
bag rather than using the same object each time. This way you do not
have to bend down continually to pick up what he dropped. I remember a father telling me that he killed two birds with one stone by using
the same object over and over again. He combined being a good dad
with his only daily exercise session. Personally, I prefer tennis.

Cause-and-effect games. It is easy to make up your own. They are extremely useful
in helping your baby learn this basic intellectual tool. When and if he is
successful, he will respond with a great sense of accomplishment. The key
to all learning is repetition. It would be unrealistic for you to expect your
baby at this age to learn a cause-and-effect concept without a great deal of
repetition. Some simple examples of cause-and-effect games are turning
the light on and off and turning a water faucet on and off. First you do it
and then you let him try, over and over again. Don't be disappointed if it

takes awhile for him to do it successfully. Yet another example of a cause-and-effect game is attaching a string to an object or toy, and then letting him have a try. When he learns to do it correctly, respond appropriately and show him how happy and proud you are.

Floor games. Too few parents get down on the floor with their babies. The floor is a fine place to get to know each other. One floor game that your baby certainly will enjoy and learn from is putting one of his familiar toys on a piece of cloth that he can grab and pull. Put the toy and cloth out of his reach and let him crawl to them. Show him how to pull the cloth so that it will bring the toy closer to him. This is an important concept, and one that he can easily learn and remember.

Hide-and-seek games. You can easily improvise any number of these games. Peek-a-boo is a favorite. Another is to cover your baby's favorite toy with a cloth or blanket and say to him, "Find the toy." If nothing happens – and it probably won't – show him the toy under the cloth or blanket and then repeat the whole process. A third idea is to put one of his balls in a box, close the cover, and say, "Find the ball." This activity will teach him how to open the box and reach in for the ball. I remember getting a call from the father of an eight-month-old boy. He was terribly upset because little Michael could not learn to open the lid of his toy box. I was even more upset with Mr. B when he told me that he raised his voice and became angry with his little boy because of this. Never frustrate or tease or get angry with your baby if he fails to accomplish a task. He feels bad enough about not being successful since he is trying his best. He must be encouraged rather than put down for his efforts.

Building and stacking games. Different-size jars or cups that fit easily inside one other are useful for these games, as are various building blocks. Again, it is important to show your baby how to build and stack while telling him in words what you are doing.

This might be a good time to reemphasize that the various recommendations I have outlined are not carved in stone. In other words, there is no reason to follow each and every one. Choose the games and activities you and your baby enjoy doing together. In our house, we particularly loved to combine wrestling and tickling. The crucial point is that positive parenting requires quality time spent with the baby. This time can be spent in your lap, in your arms, next to him in his infant seat, or on the floor together. The actual number of minutes or hours you spend is not nearly as important as the way you spend the time. That brain inside your baby's head is ready, willing, and able to absorb, learn, and develop. It is up to you to furnish the necessary stimuli, tools, and encouragement.

Nine to Twelve Months

These three months are an exciting time for your baby and a tiring time for you. The early exploratory phase (six to nine months) has passed, and now the real fun begins. I call this the Four C's Phase:

1. Curiosity
2. Crawling
3. Climbing
4. Cruising

The result of all this activity leads to a very tired parent more often than not. In addition, this period can easily become a time of stress and anxiety for all concerned. If your baby is not watched every single minute as she happily cruises and climbs all over the house, a serious accident may occur. I will never forget what a mother of a frisky ten-and-a-half-month-old girl once told me: "Would you believe that I found Barbara sitting on top of the stove with a big grin on her face. She got there by climbing up on a chair. I just never realized that she was so agile and could climb so skillfully." Luckily, dinner was not being prepared at that time. After a full day of watching and chasing after an active baby, it isn't surprising that a mother becomes exhausted, tense, and upset. A working mother coming home after a hard day at the office may also find it difficult to muster up the strength and enthusiasm to keep up with her baby.

Your baby's remarkable advances in motor skills now include being able to focus on the world of objects around her and the improving ability to transfer these objects from one hand to the other as well as the highly developed skill of being able to pick up even the smallest item (pincer movement of the fingers). The pincer movement is an important milestone in her development. A delay in acquiring this skill beyond ten months of age should be brought to the attention of her doctor. In addition, she is beginning to learn about the characteristics of objects: their shape, size, and what they can do. Can it roll or not, is it heavy or light, smooth or rough, hot or cold? And, of course, everything she gets her hands on goes right into her mouth.

A number of studies have shown that groups of children who do poorly academically in elementary school did not test out poorly (in intelligence, motor ability, language, and social development) at one year of age. It is not until two years of age that these deficits begin to be noted with testing. Despite this, most authorities on infant and early childhood development agree that these poor achievers are started on that road because they lacked proper stimulation during the first year of life. I am convinced that this nine- to twelve-month period of a baby's life is crucial in terms of her future achievement, both educationally and emotionally. Based on my experience and the experience of many others, it is clear that the extra effort you put in before your baby reaches her first birthday is very important for her subsequent intellectual and social development. Let me add that these three months are also crucial to her future physical well-being. I will discuss this in detail in the section on physical development.

Another major advance seen during these three months is the real beginning of language learning. Some babies may actually say their first meaningful words, and this is a time for celebration. On the other hand, there is really no reason to worry if your baby has not said a single recognizable word by the time she is eating a piece of her first birthday cake.

MYTH: The earlier a baby talks, the smarter she is. Or: Late talking is a sign of below-average intelligence.

Not true. There is absolutely no correlation between the age at which a baby starts to talk and her future intellectual capacity. A good example of this is my brother. Among other things, he has been a professor of electrical engineering at M.I.T. and a computer specialist who, according to our mother, did not say a meaningful word until just before age two. Of much greater significance is that your baby understands the meanings of words and sentences and the association of words with their properties (see the growth and development charts). Between nine and twelve months of age, most babies who may or may not say any words understand quite a bit of what you say.

You will notice that your baby is now beginning to realize that older people can be called upon for help. Although babies at this stage cannot yet verbalize their wants, they are able to ask for assistance by gesturing, babbling, pointing, and shouting. Those parents who are attuned and interested can easily recognize what their baby wants most of the time.

A unique aspect of this time is the long periods of time your baby spends just staring at various objects. I recall a mother asking me about her eleven-month-old, who simply stared for minutes on end at the stove, "What do you think she is thinking about?" Jokingly, I told her that Caroline was destined to become a great chef. Actually, she grew up to be an architect, and a pretty good cook besides. Obviously I could not answer her but I was pleased that she realized that her baby could, in fact, think. It is important always to remember that babies can think.

Most babies at this age continue to be quite friendly and cheerful. They love to be hugged and held and kissed, and some learn to kiss you back. You should be prepared, however, for the beginning of negative behavior. Many nine- to twelve-month-olds become stubborn and less cooperative. These traits frequently show up when they are taking a bath or when food is put on their plates. It is foolish to take this behavior personally. Your baby is not trying to upset and antagonize you. This negative streak is to be expected and should be considered perfectly normal behavior at this age.

Along with the onset of negative behavior comes teething. Teething can cause many babies a good deal of pain and discomfort, so besides being uncooperative and pig-headed, your baby may also be cranky and uncomfortable. The usual sequence for the deciduous or baby teeth to erupt is as follows: The two lower central incisors (bottom center of the mouth) come in at around six to seven months of age, and the four upper central incisors appear somewhere between seven and twelve months. When this sequence is not followed, there is no reason to be upset. I guarantee that your baby will end up with her full complement of twenty baby teeth sooner or later.

MYTH: A delay in teething is related to retarded development.

There is no correlation between the age the teeth break through and future development or intelligence. A twelve-month-old with bare gums has just as good a chance of winning the Nobel Prize as one with six teeth in place.

Before moving on to the growth and development charts, let me again remind you that the primary caretaker, whether mother, father, or somebody else, remains the key to your baby's positive development. Your baby learns most from the person who spends most of the time with her. She watches the primary caretaker for approval, to see what she can or cannot do, and for language learning. But it is also true that she can relate to and learn from more than just one primary caretaker. Aside from any surrogate who takes care of the baby for whatever reason, both mother and father ideally should function as co-primary caretakers. In my experience, a baby who is blessed with both a mother and father who practice quality parenting has the best chance to achieve her maximum potential, emotionally, intellectually, and physically. By the time the candles are lit for her first birthday party, she will be well on her way along the right road.

GROWTH AND DEVELOPMENT

PHYSICAL (MOTOR)

9-10 MONTHS

1. Stands with little or no support.
2. Walks a few steps holding on.
3. Climbs up and down from a low chair.
4. Can now sit down from a standing position.
5. Can carry two objects in one hand.
6. Adept at transferring objects from one hand to another.
7. Skillful use of "pincer" movement.
8. Cruises along furniture.

10-11 MONTHS

1. Stands alone.
2. Begins to climb stairs.
3. Walks with only a little support, holding one hand.
4. Begins to pull socks off.
5. Able to use a spoon to feed herself and to splatter the walls.
6. Can hold a crayon or a pencil and scribble with it.
7. Picks up tiny objects.

11-12 MONTHS

1. Walks alone, a few steps.
2. Climbs up and down stairs.
3. May climb out of playpen or crib.
4. Helps undress herself.
5. Handles crayon or pencil more skillfully.
6. Still prefers crawling rapidly around the house.
7. Goes from standing to sitting easily and speedily.

Note: These charts are based on average ranges of growth and development; many normal babies perform and achieve either sooner or later than indicated.

GROWTH AND DEVELOPMENT

EMOTIONAL (SOCIAL)

9–10 MONTHS

- Imitates various facial expressions and different sounds.
- Shows signs of jealousy, especially of other children.
- Well-attuned to approval and disapproval from her audience.
- Looking for fun and attention, e.g., taking off her shirt and putting it back on over and over again.
- Becoming protective of her various possessions.
- Rapid mood changes, from happy to sad to hurt to angry to cranky.
- Afraid of unfamiliar places.

10–11 MONTHS

- Enjoys music and rhythmic sounds.
- Becomes very dependent on her mother or primary caretaker.
- Less cooperative and more stubborn.
- Understands meaning of "no."
- Learns to tease parents to gain attention.
- Continually seeking approval.
- Enjoys being hugged and cuddled, and hugs back.
- Expresses many emotions and understands them in others.

11–12 MONTHS

- Good understanding of self, has learned that she's a separate and distinct person.
- Upset when separated from mother or primary caretaker.
- Fears strangers and new places.
- Negative behavior, including temper tantrums and being uncooperative, especially with eating.
- Emotionally labile: switches moods rapidly and often without any apparent reason.
- Recognizes various emotions in the people around her.
- Developing excellent sense of humor.
- Becoming more selective in activities and who she relates to.

Note: These charts are based on average ranges of growth and development; many normal babies perform and achieve either sooner or later than indicated.

GROWTH AND DEVELOPMENT

MENTAL (INTELLECTUAL)

9-10 MONTHS

- May say a word or two such as "mama" or "dada" and understand it.
- Starts to carry out simple commands such as, "Give me the ball."
- May reach for an object without actually seeing it, e.g., for a doll that is behind her.
- Begins to understand the concept of space, e.g., realizes that an object that is moved can be moved back.
- Starts to differentiate the various properties of objects, e.g., throws a ball, shakes a rattle, builds blocks, crumbles paper.
- Starts associating words with gestures, e.g., say "bye-bye" and baby waves.

10-11 MONTHS

- Begins to understand the meaning of many words. May say a couple of simple words.
- Efficient at imitating gestures and expressions of others.
- May be able to point to various parts of her body.
- Starts to associate meanings of words and their properties, e.g., bird and the sky, or a dog and barking.
- Can place small objects into a container and remove them.
- Can look for hidden objects.
- Looks at pictures in a book and begins to turn pages, usually a few at a time.
- Can pull off socks and untie shoelaces.

11-12 MONTHS

- May be able to say a few words and understand their meanings.
- Babbles short, unintelligent sentences.
- Memory improving; remembers past experiences for longer periods of time.
- Becomes involved in problem solving by trial and error.
- Can build a tower of two or three blocks.

(CONTINUED)

- Increased understanding of the association of words with their properties, e.g., say "airplane," and she looks at the sky.
- Understands meaning of more and more words and short sentences.
- Starts to group objects by class, e.g., by size or shape or color.
- Can carry out a number of different simple commands.
- Learns to find hidden objects.

Note: These charts are based on average ranges of growth and development; many normal babies perform and achieve either sooner or later than indicated.

PHYSICAL (MOTOR) DEVELOPMENT
NUTRITION

A baby who has been breast-fed up until now certainly can continue on breast milk until she reaches one year of age or even older. If during this period you decide to stop breast-feeding, I suggest that you switch over to one of the commercially prepared infant formulas. This is in keeping with the recommendation of the Committee on Nutrition of the American Academy of Pediatrics. Their recommendation is to use formula rather than cow's milk until the baby has reached one year of age.

If you have been feeding your baby formula for the first nine months, continue until one year of age. If you are breast-feeding, continue to give a daily multi-vitamin with iron. Following these recommendations will prevent your child from becoming iron-deficient. This important subject will be discussed in the next chapter, Twelve to Eighteen Months. What you should know now is that iron deficiency is associated with impaired mental development and higher blood lead levels and so it is most important to prevent iron-deficiency. A number of recent investigations have demonstrated that a baby who is iron-deficient absorbs more lead from the environment than a baby who is not iron-deficient. Lead in the blood causes severe brain damage, so it is important to keep your child's blood level as low as possible. You can't do much about the lead in the environment but you can very easily prevent your infant from becoming iron-deficient, which will help lower his blood lead level. There is further discussion on lead poisoning in the following chapter.

What about solid foods?

Babies at this age should be introduced to a variety of nutritious foods one by one. Always wait a few days after starting the baby on a new food to make certain that she can tolerate it. Your baby should be offered three well-balanced meals each day. Many babies are introduced to some regular table foods during this period, while others prefer only strained or junior foods. As I stated earlier, salt and sugar should not be added to her foods. Your child's food preferences and eating patterns are being established, and this should always be uppermost in your mind as you prepare her meals. A nutritious food that you should introduce at this time, if you have not already done so, is yogurt, preferably plain. Many adults find plain yogurt very tart and prefer it with added fruits, but your baby may well enjoy it just as it is. There is no reason to assume automatically that your baby requires the yogurt to be sweetened.

There is one aspect of nutrition that upsets many parents at this time, and that is the fact that many babies suddenly rebel against food. The battle lines are drawn. Mother does everything in her power to force the food down her baby's throat. Baby in turn does everything in her power to refuse to eat, spitting the food out or pushing it away. Through the years, I have received innumerable frantic phone calls from distraught mothers complaining bitterly about this problem. My stock answer is that I have yet to see a baby starve when food is available. A favorite story from my collection concerns a phone call from the mother of an eleven-month-old boy. She was extremely upset because Joseph stopped drinking his juice. "Dr. Eden, what should I do? If this goes on much longer, I am sure he will get scurvy." In all my years in practice, I have yet to see my first case of scurvy.

The important point to remember is that it is normal for many nine- to twelve-month-olds to develop a marked decrease in appetite. The reason is that growth is slowing down so less food is required at this time. If you understand and expect this to happen, you will be able to stop worrying about it. More about picky and finicky eaters in the next chapter.

At this age, a number of babies can hold and manipulate a cup and a spoon. Some babies like to feed themselves, even the whole meal. Others like to feed themselves only so-called "finger foods" such as crackers, pieces of banana, and cheese. Still others prefer to sit back and have you do all the work. By one year of age many babies are pretty adept at spoon-feeding themselves. I encourage you to allow your baby to feed herself even though she may make a mess of the entire feeding area.

What is really most important is allowing your baby to eat as much or as little as she wants rather than as much as you think she needs. Mealtimes for the nine- to twelve-month-old should be relaxed and cheerful, free of tension and stress. As a matter of fact, this concept holds true for any age. Unfortunately, this often is not the case. Within reason, leave the choice of foods to your baby. If a well-balanced meal is placed on her plate, the chances are good that she will choose just what her body needs over the long run. This is not simply wishful thinking on my part. A famous experiment was carried out by Dr. Clara Davis on a group of one-year-olds who were allowed to choose freely from a variety of nutritious foods. During the course of the study there was absolutely no adult involvement in the feeding. The results were astonishing. The babies ended up eating a perfectly well-balanced diet over the period of the experiment.

What do I mean by a well-balanced diet? This is a diet that contains daily servings from each of the four basic food groups:

1. Meat: includes meat, poultry, and fish, with alternative of eggs, dried beans, and soy beans
2. Vegetables and fruit: includes all fruits and vegetables
3. Milk: includes milk, cheese, yogurt, and various milk products.
4. Breads and cereals: includes breads and cereals that are whole-grained, enriched or restored; also includes rice and pasta

It makes no difference at which meal these foods are given. The important point is that your baby should be offered a variety of nutritious foods from all of these four basic food groups each day.

I will discuss between-meal snacks and so-called "junk foods" in detail in a later chapter. But as far as your nine- to twelve-month-old is concerned, let me point out that you should not fall into the trap of giving your baby unhealthy snacks when she is cranky or bored. This will start a bad habit that will be difficult to break later on. Just think about how many of us, as adolescents and adults, go on eating binges when we feel sorry for ourselves or are frustrated. The axiom to keep in mind is that food should never be substituted for love. Instead of feeding your baby when she is irritable and cranky, give her a kiss or play a game with her.

EXERCISE

There is no problem with the great majority of nine- to twelve-month-olds when it comes to physical exercise. Rather, usually the problem is trying to slow them down. With all their crawling, cruising, and climbing triggered by their great continuing curiosity, these little babies tone up and develop their muscles and coordination from morning until night. All your baby needs is the space and opportunity, and her adventurous spirit will do the rest. One of the consequences of this great amount of physical activity is an increased risk of accidents, and the prevention of accidents at this age will be covered in the section on safety tips later in this chapter.

However, there is a group of babies who do not follow this pattern of physical activity. Some nine- to twelve-month-olds are more placid, less active, and content to sit around a good deal of the time, drinking excessive amounts of milk and apple juice, munching happily on cookies and the like. It is true that some of this behavior pattern may be genetic, but I believe that most of it is due to improper parenting. Many of these basically sedentary babies are already fat, having been overfed and overstuffed from day one. The vicious cycle has started. It really does not matter which came first, the obesity or the inactivity. The fatter the baby, the more inactive she becomes. And so if your baby is obese – and you don't have to weigh her to know it; just look at her and it will be obvious – do something about it right now. Talk to her doctor about it. Cut down on the quantity of fattening foods (usually the so-called "junk foods") such as sugary cookies and make greater efforts to get her moving out of her infant seat or playpen. Offer her a piece of apple rather than a chocolate-chip cookie.

Another factor that may lead to a sedentary baby is overprotection and over concern with her physical well-being. In my experience, mothers are more often guilty of this than fathers. Parents lose sight of the long-term damage they are inflicting on the physical as well as emotional development of their baby. By continually discouraging physical activity because of the fear of an accident, parents inadvertently discourage the natural curiosity that is so crucial to healthy development. I once made a house call to see a one-year-old who had a fever and severe respiratory infection. As I walked in, I was immediately struck by the immaculately clean house, with no clutter or mess, no toys on the floor, and everything neatly in place. After examining Christina and advising Mrs. S. about treatment for the illness, I asked her if her house was always so neat. "Absolutely; I pride myself on keeping a clean and tidy house," she answered. From my point of view I would have been happier to see a messy, cluttered, lived-in house, which is to be expected with a ten-month-old baby around. Incidentally, Christina was markedly over-weight and inactive.

My advice is to not curtail your baby's desire to explore and roam. Accidents can be prevented by removing objects that might be dangerous to the baby and those she can easily destroy. For some mysterious reason, many babies at this age are fascinated by stairways. During this period, if given the chance, some learn to navigate the stairs, both up and down. This is certain-ly good exercise, but if not carefully supervised, can also be pretty danger-ous. A simple gate blocking the stairway when you are not around or unavailable to participate in this splendid activity may be the solution.

It is important to take your baby outdoors as often as you can. She will welcome the change and have more opportunities to exercise her sturdy legs and body. Many nine- to twelve-month-olds walk with a little support, and such an activity is encouraged. Less carrying around, fewer trips in the car-riage or stroller, and more walking pay off later on in helping her become more active and agile. Discouraging babies from moving around helps lead to an inactive and sedentary lifestyle later on.

Please remember that babies are sturdy and strong, and love to be han-dled and engage in roughhouse activities. Besides being a great source of pleasure, wrestling and tumbling around develop and strengthen all their muscles. These little girls and boys are not nearly as fragile as you might believe, and they need not be handled with extreme care and caution. Obviously, sensible limits should be set to avoid an accident.

There are games and materials that will help your baby's physical development. From the following list you can see that it is not necessary to buy any special equipment or apparatus.

"Go get it" games. These will be discussed in detail in the mental development section.

Hide-and-seek games. These are all good exercise and give a baby practice in moving around, whether it's crawling or cruising and occasionally walking. Many variations can be tried. For example, finger dexterity can be developed by wrapping a toy in a piece of paper and then showing your baby how to get the toy out. As the baby tires of one hide-and-see game, try another.

Pots and pans (and various sturdily constructed toys). One of the activities fascinating to most babies between nine and twelve months is banging, and although this can be pretty noisy, it is fine exercise. Elizabeth was eleven months old when her mother told me about her loud, rhythmic banging together of two favorite pots for long nonstop sessions. "You know, Dr. Eden, she practices every single day. There is no question in my mind that I'm raising the first great female drummer."

Balls. Various-sized balls, all large enough not to be swallowed or cause choking, are great fun. Footballs are a favorite since they bounce in all sorts of directions. Besides chasing the ball, your baby starts learning to throw the ball and even sometimes to catch it. This is important since instilling skills in sports is an integral part of achieving maximum physical well-being throughout life. This concept will be discussed at greater length in subsequent chapters.

SAFETY TIPS

You must now really be on the alert to prevent injuries from accidents. Statistics show that more and more unintentional injuries occur as the baby navigates around the house, crawling, cruising, and climbing.

Poisons and drugs. These must always be kept not only out of reach but out of sight. Liquor, cigarettes, furniture polish, laundry detergents, and the like all can seriously hurt or even kill your baby. So can common drugs such as aspirin, Tylenol, and Motrin if taken in large enough quantities. If you remember that babies at this age are naturally curious and adventuresome and that everything they grab goes directly into their mouths, you will act accordingly. It is good practice to always use child-safe packaging for all medicines, and have a first-aid booklet on hand for emergencies.

Automobile. You may be getting tired of hearing about this, but you must continue to use a car seat facing backward in the back seat until she weighs at least twenty pounds and is one year old. Injuries from automobile crashes are a great danger to your baby. Most serious injuries and deaths caused by car crashes would be prevented by using car safety seats every time a child is in the car. The safest place for all infants and children to ride is in the back seat. Set a proper example for your baby by using an appropriate seat belt yourself every single time you drive your car.

Burns. Nine- to twelve-month-olds grab at everything, so never carry hot liquids or hot food near your child. Don't leave cups of coffee or tea on tables or counter edges. Don't allow her to crawl around stoves or hot appliances. A safe place for your baby while you are cooking, eating, or unable to give her your full attention is in her playpen, high chair, or crib. If she does get burned, immediately put cold water on the burned area and cover with a bandage or clean cloth and call her doctor. Another good tip from the injury prevention program of the American Academy of Pediatrics to avoid severe scalding is to reduce the temperature of your hot water to between 120° F. and 130° F.

Falls. There is no way to avoid falls, but you can help prevent serious injuries by taking simple safety measures. Place gates across stairways and lower the crib mattress as your baby starts to stand. I remember two serious falls that occurred the same day. One happened to a ten-month-old boy who climbed out of his crib and landed on his head with a resultant concussion. The other was an eleven-month-old girl who fell down half a flight of stairs. Luckily, neither of these babies was seriously hurt, but your child may not be as fortunate. Always remember that the biggest threat to your baby's life and health is an unintentional injury.

Window guards should be installed on all windows above the first floor.

Dangerous objects. Since your baby is now always on the move, exploring and learning, it is necessary to keep a step ahead of her. Objects such as knives, scissors, razors, and breakables must be put away. Play areas must be cleared of sharp-edged furniture. This advice may seem obvious to you. Maybe so, but I have treated too many injuries involving such objects to take anything for granted.

Bathrooms. Babies love to play with and in water at this age – in the toilet, bathtub, or sink. Never leave your bay alone near water, even for a second. Let me again remind you that it doesn't take very long to drown.

Smoking. Although I cautioned you earlier on smoking, I want to emphasize the dangers by repeating my warnings here. Be careful with lighted cigarettes; they can very easily start a fire. Better yet, try to stop smoking altogether. You might be motivated to give this a try if you are aware of a number of studies that have proven there are more frequent hospitalizations and doctor visits during the first year for babies living in houses where the adults smoke than among babies living with nonsmoking parents. These serious illnesses are usually respiratory diseases such as pneumonia and bronchitis, and it takes very little imagination to figure out why. Cigarette smoke is not only harmful to the smoker but causes extra trouble for the baby breathing in the polluted air.

Electrical Outlets. Cover all electrical outlets with safety plugs. It is never too early to start to "child-proof" your house. This subject will be discussed in detail in the next two chapters.

Sleep. The key to both you and your baby getting a good nights sleep is to teach your baby to fall asleep on his own, without you being around. This is easier said than done. There are a number of methods that can be used, from "cold turkey" to a more gradual approach. I would suggest you discuss this with your child's pediatrician. Whatever method you choose, the principles remain the same. Your baby must learn to fall asleep on his own. The longer you postpone this, the harder it will be to succeed.

EMOTIONAL (SOCIAL) DEVELOPMENT

As I already stated and will continue to emphasize throughout the book, your goal should be a happy, well-adjusted child. Such a person has a much better chance of becoming a well-adjusted adult. You, the parents, are the key to whether she will grow up emotionally healthy and with an intact sensitivity or emotionally maladjusted with blunted sensitivity. All of us want a cheerful, contented baby who will continue that way as she grows up. None of us relish the thought of raising a baby who will turn out to be a spoiled, self-centered, nasty, and angry individual. Your approach, input, and attitude now will in large measure determine which direction your baby's emotional and social development takes.

You can expect some or all of the following normal emotional developmental milestones (listed in more detail in the growth and development charts earlier in this chapter).

1. Start of negative behavior – less cooperative and more stubborn
2. Temper tantrums
3. Emotional lability (rapid mood changes)
4. Stronger preferences for certain people and activities
5. Great dependency on the primary caretaker, and feeling upset at separation from same
6. Craving for approval and attention
7. Teasing behavior

SPECIFIC RECOMMENDATIONS

Keeping these characteristics in mind, here are some guidelines that I believe will give your baby the best chance of turning out emotionally sound:

Trusting approach. I purposely put this at the top of the list because it is the most important. What I mean by this is to approach your baby in a way that is both trusting and accepting, and in harmony with her emotional needs. If you believe in and accept the concept that your little girl is immature and totally dependent on you and that your role as parent is to meet her needs, the rest is easy. It is normal for your baby to turn to you for help and you should be happy if she does.

On the other hand, if you perceive your baby as being selfish and demanding by nature (the distrustful approach), it becomes much more difficult to satisfy her emotional needs. It is sad but true that many parents are certain that their babies are devious, cunning, and manipulative, and so "giving in" to their needs will truly lead to "spoiling" the baby. If reading this convinces you that such an attitude on your part will result in conflict, frustration, stress, and emotional injury, we will be off to a fine start.

Mrs. S. made a special appointment to talk to me about one-year-old Janet and her antisocial behavior and temper tantrums. "It seems as if I am spending most of every day punishing Janet for not behaving like a little lady" were the exact words this distraught mother used in starting our discussion. It took me three separate thirty-minute sessions to start improving this unhealthy, stressful home situation. Nine- to twelve-month-olds are not "little ladies" or "little gentlemen," and to expect them or try to force them to behave or obey is ridiculous. This family moved to Texas shortly after our talks, so I don't know how it all turned out.

Your job is not to punish inconsiderate antisocial behavior, but rather to simply discourage such behavior and encourage your baby's abilities to regulate her own actions. Sometimes, this is very difficult to do at this age so don't get discouraged. Remember the old saying, "Rome wasn't built in a day."

Overindulgence. It is easy to carry your trusting behavior too far because you are afraid of frustrating or antagonizing your baby. Don't confuse trust and acceptance with overindulgence. I am not for a minute advocating over-permissiveness, chaos, and anarchy. A certain amount of firmness is necessary for the future emotional development of your child. If things start getting out of hand, the most effective method of teaching your baby is to distract her or, if that does not work, to remove her from the unacceptable situation. The rules of acceptable behavior must be defined and explained. It is important to remember to be as consistent as possible. There is nothing more confusing and emotionally damaging for a little child than inconsistency in your responses to her actions. My favorite illustration of this confusion involved a couple whose eleven-month-old boy was a dynamo. Bobby's greatest pleasure in life was climbing up and down the stairs. Mama was continually frightened for his safety and Papa was proud of Bobby's accomplishment. You can imagine the tension in the house and the problem Bobby faced as he tried to figure out what was going on. This one turned out to be an easy one to solve. I simply advised these parents to purchase and install a movable gate across the stairs, and all was well. I could add that Bobby became a mountain climber but it wouldn't be true.

Goals. Avoid setting unrealistic goals. This is one suggestion that holds true for children of all ages and it is the one I worry about most as I write this book. It is one of the most important keys in helping your baby develop the emotional backbone and positive self-image that will stay with her forever. You do a great disservice to your baby by pushing her too hard and too fast in your frantic efforts to make her a superchild. Coercive teaching, the too-early emphasis on learning, should be discouraged. You may suspect that you are setting unrealistic goals if your baby does not enjoy the activities you introduce. If she is happy with a particular activity, the chances are good that it is the right activity for her at that time.

Restrictions. Within reason, keep restrictions to a minimum. Playpens, seats, and gates all have their place in the overall scheme of things, but they should be used judiciously. Too many restrictive devices lead to boredom and a waste of time that your baby should be enjoying. If you find that you are saying "no" and "don't touch" all day long, something is wrong. It may well be that you are not giving your baby her fair share of freedom.

Sleep. The key to both you and your baby getting a good night's sleep is to teach your baby to fall asleep on her own, without you being around. This is easier said than done. There are a number of methods, from "cold turkey" to a more gradual approach. I would suggest you discuss this with your child's pediatrician. Whatever method you choose, the principles remain the same. Your baby must learn to fall asleep on her own. The longer you postpone this, the harder it will be to succeed.

Privacy. This can be a difficult concept to understand. It has been my experience that mothers and fathers often believe that they should spend as much time as possible interacting and playing with their babies. Within certain limits they are correct. But it is just as important to realize that the baby also needs some time for herself without your active involvement. An integral part of her emotional stability is for her not to become over-dependent and over-possessive of you. Your baby should be given opportunities to play with her toys and be with her own thoughts without you always around. When she is content and happy with her privacy, you should be happy for her. Take pride in having helped her achieve this significant degree of emotional maturity at such an early age. "Can you believe it, sometimes Amy actually prefers playing with her toys to playing with me?" an upset mother reported to me one afternoon during the well-baby visit. I was very happy to hear her tell me this.

Curiosity. This remains terribly important and so it will be repeated and reemphasized. Always keep in mind that your baby must be given every opportunity to satisfy her insatiable curiosity. Many studies have shown that babies who are given the freedom to explore turn out not only more emotionally secure but do better in their academic pursuits later on.

Rewards. Reward your baby's accomplishments. This is obvious, but the way to do it may not be so obvious. The most effective method of rewarding accomplishment is with a hug and a kiss and with the right words and tone of voice. "I am so proud of you" is what I like to hear and your baby likes to hear. A reminder: rewarding accomplishment with food is discouraged. Food should not be equated with love. More about this in later chapters.

Talk. The more, the better. Most nine- to twelve-month-old babies have a very limited or no intelligible vocabulary, but they are beginning to understand the meaning of more and more words. Remember, besides what you say, your tone of voice is really what counts.

Toys and games. These will be covered in the following section on mental development. The only one I will mention now is a so-called "busy-bath" toy, of which a number of types are on the market. During this age period almost all babies have a strange fascination with water play, and such a toy serves as a continuous source of pleasure and entertainment for them.

Anything that makes your baby happy strengthens her emotional and social stability.

MENTAL (INTELLECTUAL) DEVELOPMENT

As I suggested at the start of this chapter, your baby's future intellectual achievements will depend in large measure on what she learns long before her first day at preschool. The foundation for her mental capabilities and accomplishments must be built now, and this requires the proper stimulation and activities that only you, a primary caretaker, can provide. Reading aloud from books appropriate to the child's age is most important. Literacy development leads to improved school performance, so keep reading to her, the more the better.

An important point to keep in mind is that imitation is an important way your baby learns. I remember when our son was about twelve months old and we found him seriously babbling away on the telephone one morning. Robert was not using a toy phone. After watching his father answer many phone calls each morning during the hour when parents called me for advice, he decided that it was time for him to do the same. He became a pediatrician so he is now able to continue using the skill he developed at age one. Your baby is now beginning to understand the meaning of more and more words. A sign of increasing intellectual capacity is her ability to associate the meanings of some words with their properties (see the growth and development charts). She also is discovering that the sounds she makes are a method of communicating with you. Memory is improving. She will make advances in problem solving almost entirely by trial and error.

The opportunities for learning are all around her, not only in the house but in the street, park, automobile, and stores. My advice is to take her out every chance you get and talk to her about what you see and what you are doing together. This is not a waste of your time and effort, even though your baby probably still will not understand a good deal of what you are describing. Your talking encourages her to imitate the sounds she hears. Make it a habit to touch whatever you are talking about if at all possible. Point out a tree, a dog, a car. This allows your baby to begin to associate the word or words you use with the object you are talking about – and that is what real understanding is all about. Your enthusiasm in showing your baby new places and demonstrating new activities will quickly rub off on her. All educators and psychologists agree that motivation and enthusiasm are both essential in order to achieve maximum intellectual academic attainment. It all starts with your ability to share the fun of learning with your baby. Allow me to remind you again that T.V. watching should not be part of your baby's life. As I pointed out in the previous chapter (Six to Nine Months), the American Academy of Pediatrics recommends zero T.V. watching at this age and I agree.

There are time when parents get carried away with their attempts to teach their babies something they consider important. The illustration that comes to mind is that of an art teacher who took her eleven-month-old daughter Abigail to the Metropolitan Museum of Art. Standing with her in front of a magnificent Rembrandt painting, Mrs. P. pointed to the painting and described its beauty, color, and design. All Abigail was interested in was crawling over to a nearby water fountain. The lesson to be learned is to expose your baby to as many new experiences and activities as possible but in the final analysis to allow your baby to decide what she is interested in. Don't force her to participate just because you think it's a good idea. When Abigail was nine she finally enjoyed the Rembrandt painting.

GAMES

Babies learn primarily through games. New games are needed to challenge their increasing awareness and intelligence. The interest your baby shows and the length of time she spends with each game or activity should indicate to you whether she is enjoying what she is doing. With success in figuring out a new game or activity her self-esteem expands and grows. I don't believe that any elaborate, expensive toys or games need to be purchased at this time. The following are some games that I believe will stimulate your baby's mental processes to the fullest:

"Go get it." This is a floor activity and permits your baby to practice her increasing skills in crawling, walking with support, or cruising. All you need is a ball. Simply roll it away out of her reach and say, "Go get the ball and bring it to Mommy" (or Daddy, as the case may be). If nothing happens, don't be discouraged, but try again. Encourage her with the proper words and overt signs of affection. In short order, most babies will get the hang of it, and some will even learn to roll the ball back to you.

The "go get it" game can be expanded and continued as you go about doing your household chores with your baby following you around. Ask her to bring you certain objects such as a towel or pan. She will learn the meaning of new words and the purpose of the object she fetched. For example, if she brought you a towel, wipe the dishes and tell her that the towel is drying the dish. At the next bath tell her that the towel is wiping her hands and face. This approach also teaches your baby about cooperation and being helpful; as she brings the object to you, say thank you and remind her that she has helped you. Of course, these little "helpers" slow you down considerably with their "help," but it's worth the extra time.

Filling and emptying. This type of game serves the dual purpose of increasing your baby's small-muscle skills as well as teaching her about the concept of space (see the growth and development charts). The object of the game is to put various objects into a container and then take them out. Show your baby how to do it, and always talk to her and explain what you are doing at the same time. This demonstration with words needs to be repeated until your baby can carry out the process by herself. Of course, make certain that there are no sharp-edged objects to cut her or tiny objects to swallow. After she learns what to do, leave her alone to practice. Many babies spend a good deal of time filling up and emptying containers, becoming more and more skillful at it, all the while babbling to themselves. Your baby may even at times say "no" to herself when she doesn't do it properly.

Hide and seek. Besides the exercise, this game teaches your baby problem solving. For example, put one of her small toys inside a box and then hide the box. She now has a two-step problem, first to find the box and then to open it and remove the toy. These little nine- to twelve-month-olds are amazing in their ability to concentrate and be very tenacious. After you hide an object, a baby won't give up until she finds it. Make certain, therefore, that you don't hide it too well or you may really frustrate and upset her. When she finally does find the hidden object, tell her how happy and proud you are of her achievement.

Peek-a-boo. All sorts of variations on this perennial favorite are possible. Cover your eyes and say, "Where did you go? I can't see you." Then cover her eyes and say, "Where did Daddy go? Gloria can't see me." This is a good teaching and learning experience since many babies at this age think that if they can't see you, you in turn can't see them.

Slot machine. All you need for this one is a pile of pennies and an empty plastic cup with a top in which you have cut a slot. This game is excellent for training hand dexterity, which will be especially helpful if your daughter's career goal is to be a Las Vegas card dealer. It also serves as a stimulus for your baby's interest in the results of her activity, such as dropping objects and then picking them up. The one problem with this game is the possibility that your baby will swallow a penny, but this is no catastrophe if she doesn't choke on it. Mrs. S. called me one evening and said her baby started with fifty pennies, and when the game was over there were forty-seven pennies in the container and two pennies on the floor. You guessed it: the missing penny was found in Jenny's poop four days later. You should stay with your child during this activity.

Blocks. Wooden blocks are fine. These blocks serve to help your baby learn the skill of building. Between nine and twelve months of age many babies are able to build up to three-block towers. They have more fun knocking over the tower than building it, and this can serve as a pleasurable activity for many hours on end.

Shopping. The modern supermarket with its shopping carts is an ideal situation for pleasurable learning. As you wheel your baby up and down the aisles in the cart, talk to her about the various foods on the shelves and encourage her to help you put them into the cart. Show her the pictures on the various cans as well as the different fruits and vegetables in the bins. For example, "Here's a tomato. It's red and soft." Come to think of it, since babies love to squeeze objects, maybe a tomato is the wrong example. A head of lettuce is a better idea. After you get home, show her what you do with the different foods you bought. Later, as she eats them, remind her about what you did together in the supermarket.

When I have the opportunity to go supermarket shopping myself, I am very interested in watching mothers with their babies. One type of mother spends all her time saying "no" and denying the baby a chance to participate, and both mother and baby usually are upset and miserable. The other type of mother involves her baby in the experience. The babies who are encouraged to participate look happier and are also learning and expanding their knowledge.

I'd like to close this chapter by exploding an old wives' tale that is unrelated to anything physical, mental, or emotional but is appropriate to this age.

MYTH: Giving a baby a haircut before one year of age brings bad luck.

I don't understand where or how this one started, but it is not true. Happy first birthday!

Twelve to Eighteen Months

"Where does he get all that energy?" I am asked this question over and over again by the parents of twelve- to eighteen-month-olds. The parents of these children are amazed by the tremendous activity level of their toddlers, on the move literally from morning until night. If you think you were tired before, during the nine- to twelve-month age, the real fun is only beginning. These little people, besides showing more independence, impulsiveness, and self-assertion, are still just as curious and adventuresome as before. Your twelve-to eighteen-month-old is beginning to make the discovery of "self." It's as if he seems to shout, "I want to do this my way, be myself, and now!" If you combine all these traits with his increased efficiency in walking and climbing, the results are obvious. But there is even more to look forward to: the start of negative behavior. The so-called "terrible twos" start earlier than age two, often some time between fourteen and eighteen months. Your youngster now understands the meaning of "no," not only your "no" but his own "no" as well. He becomes stubborn and less cooperative and may refuse to obey your requests or demands. He will also do his best to take over. The result becomes a real test of wills. What I am describing is normal behavior for a baby of this age and so it is best that you be prepared for it. Do not take it personally, and remember that this too will pass.

Your toddler should be sleeping about thirteen hours per day, including an afternoon nap. The bedtime ritual should include a warm bath, reading a favorite picture book, hugs and kisses, and perhaps a night light. Try not to deviate from this routine.

Your baby is now able to explore the whole world around him quickly and efficiently. Since he now stands a good deal of the time he can see much more than he could before. He can see tabletops and all the objects on them, bookshelves, television knobs, computers, and all the other fascinating items in his environment. This widening of his horizons is new, interesting, and exciting for him but it creates additional problems for you, especially relating to his safety and the safety of your possessions. At this point you have two basic choices, and the one you make (consciously or unconsciously) will in large measure determine whether you will be successful in achieving the goal of this book – helping your child develop to his maximum potential now and later on in life. You can either basically keep your house for the adults in it or you can "child-proof" it for your baby. If you don't follow any other suggestions I make please follow this one: child-proof your house! (Specific guidelines and recommendations as to how to do so are listed in the safety section later on in this chapter.) Your toddler needs plenty of room and opportunity to play. Dr. Jean Piaget, the famous Swiss psychologist, one of the true pioneers in infant and early child development, describes this period as the phase of experimentation. The insatiable curiosity your baby shows should always be encouraged. This approach will surely make him more successful and self-confident later on in school and in his chosen occupation. If his curiosity is squelched at every turn because you are afraid of accidents or the destruction of your possessions, it will lead to lowered self-confidence and an increase in self-doubt, and these traits may well stay with him throughout his school years and beyond.

All educators agree that success in school is based on the following four factors:

1. Verbal confidence
2. Problem-solving ability
3. Independence, curiosity, and enthusiasm
4. Sociability and control of emotions

These next six months of your baby's life are critical to achieving these goals. Each will be covered in detail in the appropriate section of this chapter.

A few words about language are in order at this point. You can expect your baby to say up to six meaningful words by the time he is eighteen months old. He will surely understand many more words and phrases and should be able to respond to simple commands such as "Give that to me" as you point to a particular object or toy. Since he learns by imitation, it is important that you speak to him slowly and clearly in a calm, quiet tone of voice. When he does say a meaningful word, do not imitate his pronunciation but rather repeat the word to him correctly.

Let me get back to the superenergy of your toddler. His increased activity takes many forms. He loves to throw food, ransack closets, open drawers and throw out everything he can get his little hands on. A mother of a sixteen-month-old described in amazement the speed and efficacy with which Andy emptied out an entire drawer full of clothes during the minute or two it took her to go downstairs to answer the doorbell. What was lovely about this mother was that she told me the story with pride and pleasure rather than with frustration and anger. These young explorers climb into toilets and onto tables and up and down stairs. Try to consider these exploits as serious experiments in his continuing thirst and quest for learning. If you accept this type of behavior as his method of learning and not as "naughty" behavior or his way of upsetting you, it will prevent a good deal of trouble, both for you and for your child. Two more examples illustrate what I mean:

Mother No. 1 reported what her fifteen-month-old had just done to her. "Dr. Eden, Joseph just crawled into the living room and smashed my most expensive piece of glassware. I am sure he did it to torture me." Mother No. 2 informed me that her seventeen-month-old boy just climbed out of his crib for the first time. "Dr. Eden, wasn't that a fantastic accomplishment? I am so proud of him." All things being equal, Jimmy, who was lucky to have mother No. 2, has a much better chance of developing to his full potential.

In my experience, many parents use the T.V. set as a baby-sitter. "You know, Dr. Eden, the only peace and quiet I have is when I sit Andy down in his highchair in front of the T.V. with some snacks." My answer to that mother was, "You may be getting some peace and quiet, but you are doing very little for Andy. One-year-olds learn nothing from T.V. except to become sedentary, lazy, and fat." That mother was not happy with my answer, which I admit could have been expressed more diplomatically. More about T.V. in later chapters.

It's easier said than done, but try to keep your "no's" to a minimum. As one mother recently told me, "I'm doing much better. I'm pretty sure I went through an entire day with less than one hundred no's." Save your no's for important occasions, such as when he's around hot stoves or open windows. If you say no to every minor infraction of the rules, your baby is less likely to pay attention to you when it really counts.

During this time you will probably notice that your child is starting "make believe" behavior, such as talking into a toy telephone or pretending to drive a toy truck. Our son was an avid transportation enthusiast at this age. He would drive all sorts of toy cars and trucks for hours on end each day.

He is now all grown up and still involved in transportation, but now he pilots a real airplane, besides being a pediatrician.

Many twelve- to eighteen-months-olds begin to show preference for one hand over the other. I would strongly advise to not interfere in any way and to not encourage using the right hand over the left. For those of you who hope that your child grows up to be a champion tennis player, this suggestion is easy to follow. After all, Rod Laver, Jimmy Connors, and John McEnroe were all left-handed and it didn't hurt their careers in the slightest. On the contrary, it probably gave them an advantage. For what it is worth, I also am left-handed. Forcing a naturally left-handed person to change may lead to learning, speech, and writing problems later on. So simply let nature take its course.

Before we move on to the growth and development charts, let me emphasize that although it will be more work for you, try to give your baby the benefit of the doubt as he roams about. He must be allowed to begin to break loose from you and become more independent and self-sufficient. He should be allowed to explore and learn, since pride in achievement is essential for his future well-being. Take a balanced approach in your parenting. By this I mean that you should not put too much emphasis on one particular area. Rather, give equal time and effort to his physical, emotional, and mental development. Most important, don't try to push him too hard or too fast. Each child develops at a different rate and no two are alike. All you have to do is love him and trust him. The time you spend with him should be quality time. Show him you're on his side and give him the space, opportunity, and tools to be active and happy.

GROWTH AND DEVELOPMENT

PHYSICAL (MOTOR)

12–15 MONTHS

- Walks with slight support or walks alone.
- Climbs onto low chairs and sofas.
- Skillful pincer movements of thumb and index finger.
- Can usually build two- to three-block towers.
- Proficient in removing small objects from receptacles.
- Can sometimes climb stars while standing and holding on, and often on hands and knees.
- Enjoys feeding himself; usually holds and handles spoon and cup.
- Can unscrew tops of cans and turn doorknobs.
- Enjoys sitting on floor and pivoting around while at play.

15–18 MONTHS

- Walks well, trots, and begins to run.
- Can scribble with a pencil or crayon.
- Fine stairway climber.
- Can stand on one foot and can walk backward.
- Can build three- to four-block towers.
- May climb out of crib.
- Throws ball with enthusiasm but with little control.
- Walks along with pull-toys.
- Can turn pages of book, usually more than one page at a time.
- Begins to show hand preference.

Note: These charts are based on average ranges of growth and development; many normal babies perform and achieve either sooner or later than indicated.

GROWTH AND DEVELOPMENT

EMOTIONAL (SOCIAL)

12-15 MONTHS

- Shows affection.
- Fine sense of humor, laughs heartily.
- Loves audiences and demands attention.
- More self-assertive and stubborn and may show signs of temper and temper tantrums.
- Begins to show real negative behavior.
- Rapid mood shifts.
- Loves to imitate, especially doing housework.
- Upset with separation from familiar people; prefers certain people over others.

15-18 MONTHS

- Starts to say no.
- Willful, stubborn, negative, with or without temper tantrums.
- Becoming less afraid of strangers.
- Still demands attention.
- Aware and sensitive to the emotions of parents; sometimes can be cooperative, e.g., hands certain objects to parents, waves bye-bye on request.

Note: These charts are based on average ranges of growth and development; many normal babies perform and achieve either sooner or later than indicated.

GROWTH AND DEVELOPMENT

MENTAL (INTELLECTUAL)

12–15 MONTHS

- Begins to use language; says up to six meaningful words.
- Understands and responds to some words and some short phrases.
- Jabbers and babbles with expression.
- Responds and comes when called.
- Imitates simple acts, such as household chores.
- Can fit blocks into appropriate-sized openings.
- Can find and bring back an object that is hidden.
- Able to point to familiar objects and people when asked.
- Can look at pictures in a book with understanding.
- Enjoys taking off some of his clothes.
- May be able to make his wishes known by gestures and voice expressions.

15–18 MONTHS

- Meaningful vocabulary, sometimes up to ten words or more, and a couple of two-word phrases such as "bye-bye" and "all gone."
- Great increase in understanding words and phrases, responds to questions, and follows simple commands.
- Calls himself by name, and his favorite word is "no."
- Excellent ability to imitate words without necessarily knowing their meaning.
- Very proficient at imitating adults' behavior and actions.
- Can point to different parts of his body on request.
- Can handle a crayon or pencil fairly well; usually scribbles but may occasionally draw a relatively straight line.
- Can put simple puzzles together.
- Avid explorer, especially of drawers, wastepaper baskets, and toilet bowls.

Note: These charts are based on average ranges of growth and development; many normal babies perform and achieve either sooner or later than indicated.

PHYSICAL (MOTOR) DEVELOPMENT

NUTRITION

The decrease in appetite seen in some nine- to twelve-month-olds may be even more dramatic during the twelve- to eighteen-month period. Many toddlers at this age become choosy and finicky eaters and develop distinct food dislikes as well as preferences. There are days when they eat next to nothing. Accept this as normal behavior. Believe me when I tell you that your child won't starve or waste away if he skips a few meals.

If you are still breast-feeding your baby and both of you are happy with it, there is no reason to stop. When you stop breast-feeding switch to regular whole cow's milk. Babies who have been on formula also can now be given regular cow's milk.

MYTH: Every child needs to drink one quart of milk per day.

This belief is great for the dairy industry, but there is no medical or nutritional reason for a child to drink a quart each day. All of us, including toddlers and children, can get along very well on considerably less. Two glasses of milk per day (a total of sixteen ounces) are enough to satisfy all your child's needs, including his calcium requirements. The current recommendations of the Committee on Nutrition of the American Academy of Pediatrics is to avoid skim or low-fat milk until the toddler is two years old, and I agree. Studies have demonstrated that the brain needs a certain amount of fat for optimal development during this period of very rapid growth. The total daily calcium requirement for a one- to three-year-old is 500 milligrams. One cup of milk contains 250 milligrams of calcium, as does one cup of yogurt. If your baby enjoys drinking milk, let him have as much as he wants, as long as you do not exceed one quart per day. Drinking more than that will interfere with his appetite for solid foods.

Your toddler should continue the well-balanced, nutritious diet that was outlined in the previous chapter. Most babies can now eat alongside the rest of the family. Many enjoy feeding themselves and become pretty skillful in handling a spoon and cup. Some need more help than others. There are those children who still prefer strained baby foods and reject the lumpier table foods. In such cases, it is perfectly acceptable to continue to feed your child baby foods. Offer him a varied diet, including plenty of fruit and vegetables. Stay away from so-called junk foods as much as possible. The subject of snacks will be discussed in the next chapter.

IRON DEFICIENCY

We all want our children to grow up as smart as possible. One foolproof way to improve your child's mental development is to prevent him from ever becoming iron-deficient. This is so simple but unfortunately many parents are just not aware of the relationship between iron-deficiency and impaired mental and psychomotor development and so unknowingly may be responsible for their children losing precious I.Q. points.

Many studies have proven beyond doubt that iron-deficiency anemia during the second year of life, the period when the baby's brain is growing rapidly, can cause damage to the developing brain. Even after the anemia is corrected, the damage to the brain remains long-lasting.

One of the true success stories in pediatrics has been the virtual elimination of iron-deficiency anemia during the first year of life. The success has mainly been due to an increase in breast-feeding and the use of iron-fortified formulas and cereals. Unfortunately, this success story is not true for many toddlers who develop iron-deficiency anemia during the second year of life and so are at risk for impaired intellectual development. The actual prevalence of iron-deficiency and iron-deficiency anemia in one- to two-year-olds in the United States is in question. Most recently studies including our own report about a ten percent incidence of iron-deficiency anemia and a thirty percent incidence of iron-deficiency without anemia. These figures show that currently there are a large number of toddlers who are iron-deficient during the second year of life.

Why are so many one- to two-year-olds iron-deficient? The following is the usual scenario that occurs at around one year of age:

1. The baby is switched from either breast milk or an iron-fortified formula to regular milk, which contains very little iron.

2. Infants cereals, iron-fortified by law in the United States, are often discontinued in favor of adult-type cereals, most of which are not iron-fortified.

3. A baby's appetite for solid foods decreases at about one year of age. Many of these toddlers become finicky eaters while drinking large quantities of whole milk and apple juice, neither of which contains iron. A recent large-scale review dealing with the nutrition of one- to two-year-olds determined that sixty percent were not receiving their recommended daily allowance of iron. As a matter of fact, surveys have indicated that this is the period (one to two years of age) during which the least amount of iron is taken in through diet as compared to any other period in life.

Making the case for iron-deficiency's effect on development even stronger was a recent study conducted by Jill Halterman and associates from the Department of Pediatrics at the University of Rochester School of Medicine. This investigation demonstrated that six- to sixteen-year-old children who were iron-deficient scored lower in math than a similar group of children who were not iron-deficient.

A second significant danger of iron-deficiency in toddlers lies in its relationship to lead poisoning. Recent studies have proven that iron-deficiency increases lead absorption. This means that toddlers who are iron-deficient have higher blood lead levels than those who are not iron-deficient. The higher the blood lead level, the more I.Q. points are lost forever. Put another way, the lower the blood lead level, the more I.Q. points are saved. Even low blood levels, previously thought to be harmless, have been shown to lower the I.Q. Dr. Bruce Lanphear and his associates at the Children's Hospital Medical Center in Cincinnati found that toddlers with blood lead levels lower than 10 mcq/dl, levels previously considered normal, in fact also caused the loss of precious I.Q. points.

With these facts in mind, any discussion of iron-deficiency must include its relationship to lead absorption. By preventing iron-deficiency you will help protect your child from increased absorption of lead from the environment. An old saying goes, "You can never be too rich or too thin." I think we should now add "or have a blood lead level too low."

I hope that by now I have convinced you of the importance of preventing iron-deficiency from ever developing in your child. The ideal method of prevention is having your child eat a diet that contains a sufficient amount of iron. Most of the time this just does not happen. I do not agree with the secondary prevention approach of the American Academy of Pediatrics. Their recommendation is only to screen for anemia at twelve months of age and treat it if the child is found to be anemic. The test that is used (hemoglobin or hematocrit) only checks for anemia and does not test for iron-deficiency.

I believe it is safer, easier, and more effective to give all babies supplemental iron when they are switched to regular whole milk. This daily supplement can be given either as an iron-fortified vitamin, iron drops, or an iron-fortified nutritional drink. In our office, we put every baby on an iron-fortified vitamin preparation when they start to drink regular milk. I strongly believe that this primary prevention approach will protect a baby from ever becoming iron-deficient. Why take a chance when it's so easy to prevent trouble? I strongly suggest that you discuss this with your baby's doctor.

Mealtimes should be pleasant and relaxed – but sad to say, often they're just the opposite. Decreased appetite, negative behavior, and over-activity can easily lead to chaos in the kitchen. If you want your child to eventually learn to eat a sensible, well-balanced, and nutritious diet, don't make his life miserable by forcing him to eat when he is not hungry. This is one recommendation that in my experience many parents find difficult to accept. I probably spend more time talking to parents about not forcing food than about any other subject, although I must admit that discussions related to the excretory functions of the baby run a close second. There is more and more evidence proving how important a well-balanced diet is for the future physical well-being of the child. Eating habits are learned early, so this is the time to establish sound eating practices.

With table foods taking the place of strained baby foods, this is the time to discuss salt and sugar. As I mentioned earlier, the leading baby-food manufacturers have stopped adding salt to all their products and sugar to all but a few. You should do the same. Make certain not to add salt or sugar when cooking and preparing table foods for your baby. If he is raised on a diet that is high in sugar and salt, he will quickly learn to enjoy these tastes and will grow up continuing to eat the same way. Let me repeat that babies are not born craving salt or sugar. These preferences are acquired.

It is estimated that the average person in the United States consumes twelve grams of salt per day, which is many times the recommended daily requirement. You may well be inadvertently starting your baby on a diet that is too high in salt when you introduce him to table foods. Many parents add more salt than necessary during cooking and add even more at the table. What happens is you prejudge your child's food-taste preferences and use your own taste buds to decide how the food should taste. I'm the perfect example of a "salt freak," and this dates back to my early childhood. My mother used to bribe me with salty foods such as olives and pickles to get me to eat my oatmeal. She later told me that since she always loved salt, she assumed that I would also. As of today, although I know better, I sprinkle salt on my hot cereal and, as a matter of fact, on almost anything I eat. You will be doing your child a great disservice if you get him used to extra salt. There is enough natural salt in foods for your baby's needs. The evidence is clear that too much salt can lead to high blood pressure and kidney disease later on, or it can aggravate or enhance the problem if a familial or underlying tendency to hypertension is present.

If your baby becomes accustomed to a lot of sugar, I can guarantee you that he will always crave it. It is frightening to think about, but according to the latest estimate, the average United States citizen swallows more than one hundred pounds of sugar per year. The less sugar you add to the foods you feed your baby, the better. There is plenty of natural sugar in our foods, so from the nutritional point of view it is not necessary to add any more. Toddlers raised on a diet without added sugar become accustomed to such a diet and enjoy and thrive on it. Besides extra unnecessary calories that can cause obesity, excess sugar promotes dental decay. Of even greater significance in terms of the long-range physical well-being of your child is the evidence that a too-high sugar intake may contribute to the future development of heart disease. Refined sugars tend to increase the triglyceride (fat) level in the blood, one of the risk factors involved in developing coronary heart disease. Babies learn by example, so it would be best if you also cut down on the amount of salt and sugar you use. If you can do so, you get an extra added bonus – your own health is bound to improve.

A final point about nutrition: A baby normally triples his birth weight by one year of age. For example, a seven pound newborn should weigh about twenty-one pounds at one year. If your baby has considerably more than tripled his birth weight, he may be overweight. If so, it is a good idea to check it out with your baby's doctor, who might choose to take certain steps to slow down your baby's weight gain. If one or both parents are overweight, it is even more important to monitor the weight of the child, since genetics plays such an important role in obesity.

The results of a large-scale survey of more than 2,800 one- to four-year-old children were published very recently. They showed that for the overweight toddlers in this group, increased servings of fruit juice were associated with excess weight gain. The study also concluded that increased amounts of whole fruit in the diet reduced weight gain. The bottom line: Cut down on the amount of juice you offer your baby. Apple juice appears to be the biggest offender. I conducted an unofficial survey in my office and found that many toddlers drink enormous quantities of apple juice each day, some as much as thirty-two ounces. My suggestion is to limit the intake of all juices to no more than six to eight ounces per day.

EXERCISE

These little dynamos, with exceptions, are naturally superactive and more than ready for all physical activity. They require the space and opportunity and need the proper toys and materials to develop both their small and large muscles to the fullest. For the first time, a purchase of some special equipment is useful, but elaborate and expensive paraphernalia is not necessary.

The following are my specific suggestions for helping to develop your baby's coordination, strength, and muscles.

Push- and pull-toys. By this I mean toys such as cars and trucks. These are great fun and give your child the opportunity to move around in his make-believe world. Many of these push- and pull-toys have noises built in to function as they move, and the sound effects make the activity even more pleasurable. These toys are useful for both small- and large-muscle development.

Balls. Let your child take the lead in playing with balls of various sizes. Some babies this age learn to throw a ball, but it is a bit too soon for you to try to teach him to pitch to a target. Footballs and ping-pong balls seem to be particularly useful.

Crawling games. Anything you can figure out that will make crawling fun for your baby is splendid exercise for his large muscles. One example would be a large cardboard box such as the box a television set comes in. Simply cut out the sides and presto – he has an indoor or outdoor playhouse.

Small-muscle activities.
1. Hammering toys: These are noisy but necessary. Your child learns dexterity and becomes better coordinated while having a great time pounding away.
2. Beads for stringing: Large wooden beads on a thick string are fine. By around eighteen months of age most toddlers are ready to play with beads. Make certain that the beads don't

break off. Since everything your baby picks up goes directly into his mouth he can easily choke on a bead.

3. Plastic snap-lock rings: These are made to be pulled apart and snapped together. Your child can spend many happy hours practicing this new skill.

Roughhouse activities. No special equipment is needed except a soft enough floor (put down a blanket or pad) or a bed. The more of these activities, the better, not only for his overall physical development but for his emotional well-being as well. The wrestling match should be interrupted frequently for rest periods and big hugs.

Chase him and catch him games. There is little question that you will get tired of these games sooner than your child will.

Hide-and-seek games. This type of game still is a favorite.

Outdoor yard play. Having your own or a neighbor's yard is ideal, but if it's not available, it is no great tragedy. A playground with the proper equipment is just as good, but in some neighborhoods such a facility is hard to find. Weather permitting, get your baby outside as often as possible. There are several types of outdoor yard play that children especially enjoy.

They love playing in a sandbox filled with plenty of dirt (be sure it is not combined with dog or cat feces). A lot of dirt is the key. I once talked to a mother of an eighteen-month-old boy whose greatest pleasure in life was rolling around in the dirt. Mrs. F. happened to be a fastidious lady who could not stand seeing Johnny dirty and so she took him out of his natural habitat every hour on the hour. She would drag him screaming and yelling into the house to give him a bath and then take him back to his sandbox. All I can say is that this little guy was pretty water-logged by dinnertime.

MYTH: Dirt is unhealthy for a child.

Nothing could be further from the truth. There is nothing dangerous about dirt as long as it is not mixed with animal feces or eaten in large quantities. A bath before dinner after a whole day of wallowing in dirt is sufficient.

Children also enjoy playing on climbing equipment. This is a real luxury but can be used well beyond eighteen months of age. There are a number of different types of climbing equipment on the market. A low-to-the-ground jungle gym is one. Another is a dome climber, based on the geodesic principle of construction developed by the famous Buckminster Fuller. It is sturdy and can hold as many kids as can climb on it at a given time. The dome climber should be set up on either grass or sand to soften and cushion any possible falls. It is well-constructed and can give good service throughout the entire preschool period. It furnishes fine exercise and also builds up your baby's self-confidence as he becomes a more proficient climber. The dome climber has another function: covered with canvas, it instantly coverts to a tent or fort.

If you have a yard, your child will also like water play. All you need is a plastic basin and some plastic toys. The important thing to remember is to keep the water level no higher than four inches. I advise that this activity always be supervised.

Indoor climber and slide. There are a number of these on the market. If you have the room and resources, one of these can function as an excellent resource for good exercise and play when weather or circumstances do not permit you to go outside with your baby.

Let me close this section by reminding you that plenty of fresh air is healthy for your child. Get him outside every chance you get. Even if he has a simple cold but is acting normally, there is no reason to keep him indoors. If he has a full-blown upper respiratory infection, it would be unfair to have him play with other children because he can spread his cold to them, but the outdoor air won't hurt him at all. Speaking of colds, here is another widely believed old wives' tale:

MYTH: Washing a child's hair or giving him a bath while he has a cold will cause pneumonia.
There is no truth to this. All you have to do is dry him thoroughly and then let him go about the normal business of the day.

SAFETY TIPS

The key is to child-proof your apartment or house. This means making a systematic, slow, and careful trip through your entire home (including the backyard, basement, and garage if you live in a house). Try to look at things through the eyes of your toddler. Ask yourself, "Is there anything dangerous lying around that he can get hold of?" If the answer is yes, remove all such objects. A baby between twelve and eighteen months cannot be expected to differentiate between what is safe and what is unsafe. I have been involved in many toddler accidents caused entirely by not properly child-proofing the house.

Poisons. Many products commonly found in the house can be poisonous. Some common examples are aspirin, sleeping pills, moth balls, bleach, cosmetics, drain cleaners, and lye. The Committee in Injury, Violence, and Poison Prevention of the American Academy of Pediatrics lists the following safety rules:

1. Keep dangerous products out of your child's sight and reach.
2. Take extra care during times of family stress.
3. Never call medicine "candy."
4. Buy medicine and household products in child-resistant packages and use these packages as directed. (Even these can be opened by many children.)
5. Never leave alcoholic beverages within a child's reach.
6. Seek help if your child has swallowed a nonfood substance.

You should also be aware of another type of poisoning caused by lead ingestion. Lead sources are everywhere in our environment. Paint is still by far the most common source of lead in the urban United States. Before 1950, most houses were painted both inside and outside with paint containing large amounts of lead. Many of these homes, which have now deteriorated, are particularly dangerous since the lead paint can be inhaled in the form of dust; also, some children eat the paint as it chips. In 1973, the United States federal government forbade the sale via interstate commerce of paint containing more than 0.5 percent lead. Nevertheless, there are still many houses with high-content-lead paint still on their walls. Plaster containing lead is also a common source. It is estimated that thirty million such dwellings are still in use, about one-quarter of which are in debilitated condition. If you live in such a house, I would advise that you immediately take the necessary precautions to eliminate this potentially serious poison. If you live in an old house, during construction or renovation, my best advice is to remove your baby from the premises. If kept at home he will breathe in lead-containing dust and with hand-to-mouth activity he will swallow the dust. Lead poisoning can cause severe irreversible brain damage. Be especially careful if your child is in the habit of eating nonfood substances (called pica). The higher the blood lead level, the greater the mental impairment. But even low lead levels have been shown to damage the developing brain of a toddler.

Falls and cuts. Always remember that doors and screens at stairways, doorways, and other dangerous areas should be safely fastened. Use plastic dishes and cups. Try to remove furniture with sharp edges and use nonskid mats in the bathtub. It is essential that you install appropriate guards on all windows, especially above the ground floor.

Drowning. Never leave your child alone in water (whether he's in the bathtub or elsewhere) since even shallow water is dangerous. You must always accompany your child to a pool or lake.

Automobile. Never allow your child to play alone in the driveway or in the car. Place safety latches on your car doors. While the car is in motion, always use an approved car restraint or seat. He can now ride facing forward provided he weighs at least twenty pounds, but he should still remain in the back seat.

Hearing. One of the main reasons for speech delay is a hearing loss and the sooner it is identified, the better the outcome. If a one-year-old does not start to imitate the sounds made to him, it is a possible danger signal pointing to a hearing problem. If this is the case with your baby, consult his doctor.

EMOTIONAL (SOCIAL) DEVELOPMENT

Let's start this section by listing some of the expected character traits of your twelve- to eighteen-month-old. With these in mind you will be in a better position to continue to help your baby develop the emotional stability and positive self-image so essential for his future well-being. You can look forward to:

1. Negative behavior
2. Impulsiveness
3. Self-assertion
4. Independence
5. Selfishness and stubbornness
6. Demands for attention
7. Rapid mood changes
8. Sense of humor
9. Affectionate behavior

As you can see, your work is cut out for you. How you handle your child during these six months will either begin to prepare him to cope with the outside world with optimism and enthusiasm or will lower his chances of growing up happy, secure, and self-reliant.

SPECIFIC RECOMMENDATIONS

The following are the specific activities, toys, and approaches that I believe will encourage your toddler to develop the positive social characteristics that you would like to see.

Other children. It is a good idea at this point to start inviting other children close to your baby's age into your house, as well as take your baby out to the park so that he can establish contact with his peers. Your baby needs the company of other children, and this will better prepare him for future nursery school and preschool experiences. Of course, if you have an older sibling around, your baby has already learned a bit about socializing and sharing, and very often, unfortunately, also about not sharing.

Sharing. Although the twelve- to eighteen-month-old is basically pretty selfish, it is nevertheless important to begin to teach him what sharing is all about. You can do this alone with him but it is more effectively accomplished when other children are around. For example, with two other playmates present, bring out three of your child's toys and distribute them, one to each child, explaining what you are doing. I must admit that this does not always work out, but it's worth a try.

Daily routine. Babies at this age are happy with a set routine and become confused and upset if each day is totally different from the previous one. Therefore, within limits, try to establish a set daily routine. Let your baby know that it's naptime or time to put away his toys; he will enjoy these rituals, and it will also help him acquire good habits.

Consistency. Your approach and responses should always be consistent. Your baby will continually test you to see if you really mean what you say. There is nothing more disturbing for the child than having you say "yes" one time and "no" the next to the same request or action on his part. Both the mother and father must try to remain consistent. But often this turns out not to be easy. Think about it, two people who grow up with different value systems now have to try to agree. If not, your baby will start playing one parent against the other, and this destructive game will only get worse as he grows older.

Protection versus overprotection. Overprotection will fill your child with needless fears, hurt his self-confidence, and lower his self-image. If you have adequately child-proofed your house, let him go and don't worry too much about his physical safety. This leads me to the subject of falls. Toddlers all fall down, usually many times a day. You can sympathize with him but unless the fall is a nasty one, my advice is not to make a big fuss. Rather than run to his aid, let your baby get up by himself. This approach will help him build up his self-confidence and independence and will reduce his overdependence on you.

Negative behavior. Don't fall into the trap of responding to your toddler's anger and stubbornness by screaming and yelling. Mrs. W. came to my office to ask my advice about handling Thomas's temper tantrums. "Would you believe that Tom actually screams and wildly kicks the wall when he does not get his way?" It turned out that little Tom had learned to kick walls from big Tom, his father, who, when sufficiently provoked, did exactly the same thing. Many of us forget the truism that children learn primarily by example.

Except for special occasions, such as when he's tried to climb out the window, try to not hit your baby, no matter how angry you are. I would also discourage you from yelling and threatening. The most effective way to handle your child's negative behavior is to distract him with a toy, another activity, or a change of scene. If all that does not work, I would suggest that you simply separate him from you, remaining calm and quiet as you do so. Put him in his room and explain to him that when he feels better about things, he can come back out. Toddlers are extremely sensitive to your emotions and will understand when you are disappointed in their behavior. Although they can't speak too well themselves, they have a clear understanding of what is going on around them.

Unrealistic goals. Do not expect or demand perfection from your baby. Rather, whenever possible, register your pride in his accomplishments. For example, if he shares his toys with a playmate, make a big fuss about it and tell him how proud you are. If he responds to one of your requests such as handing you something you ask for, give him a big kiss and a hug and tell him how happy you are that you have him. It is a two-way street: you are around to make him happy and he must also learn that he is around to make you happy.

Exploration. Give your child opportunities to explore and learn. If he somehow gets his hands on one of your favorite books and tears out every single page, don't react as if this is hostile on his part. Although it won't be easy, accept it as his only way of learning a new skill, part of his scientific research for that day.

Rules. At this age you should begin to teach your toddler some simple rules and routines, such as touching people gently. Again, praise him when he does follow the rules.

TOYS

Dolls and cuddly soft animals. These encourage feelings of tenderness, protection, and care and are very important. They are also useful in helping your baby with dramatic play. He will be able to act out more easily the rules of various family members and will also be better able to play out important emotions. It's a good idea to store these dolls and large soft animals on a shelf that your child can reach by himself when he wants them.

MYTH: Little boys who play with dolls will turn out to be homosexual.

I am glad to say that nowadays fewer parents believe this. Similarly, little girls who play with trucks don't turn out to be lesbians. Little boys should be allowed to play with dolls and little girls with trucks, and in the end it all works out fine.

Mr. J. called me one morning, bitterly complaining about the doll his little boy received as a birthday present from Mr. J.'s mother-in-law. "What's she trying to do, make Mike a fairy?" I happened to be in a particularly cranky mood that day, so I told him what I thought about this in rather strong terms.

Rhythm instruments. Drums, cymbals, tin cans, and metal pans are all useful, and your toddler will enjoy playing with them. Even though you and your neighbors may not appreciate the noise, it is wrong to deprive him of this pleasurable activity.

Music. Twelve- to eighteen-month-olds have broad musical tastes. They love to dance in time to the music, either by themselves or with you. They also love rhymes and jingles and are good at imitating. Incidentally, music is a fine way to improve a nasty mood. As I am writing this section, I'm listening to Mozart and my mood is improving minute by minute.

I would be remiss if I did not warn you about an interesting trait that is common during this twelve- to eighteen-month period: sudden silence. I advise you to immediately stop whatever you are doing and go investigate. The chances are good that he has found something extremely interesting to occupy his time. Here is one example that comes to mind: Mrs. P. told me about the time her seventeen-month-old had quietly smeared an entire living room wall with her red lipstick. "I found my little painter standing in front of the wall silently admiring his artwork with a great big smile on his face." How would you have reacted to this? Another example of the "sudden silence" syndrome took place in the bedroom. That little guy didn't use lipstick. His walls were painted brown.

MENTAL (INTELLECTUAL) DEVELOPMENT

During these six months your baby will make tremendous advances in his intellectual capacities. His memory is improving day by day. He imitates more and more efficiently without actually understanding the meaning of most of the words or phrases he imitates. He will become more and more interested in pictures and he will start to solve simple puzzles. Most important is that his understanding of the world around him and his verbal comprehension both expand enormously. It is important to remember that repetition is still the key to his learning.

As yet he probably will not be able to internalize his thinking process. The "thoughtfulness" that is characteristic of a baby over eighteen months of age is usually not seen. A child younger than eighteen months attempts possible solutions before trying to solve the problem. Rather, he jumps right in, using trial and error instead of pausing or taking the time to evaluate the situation. Come to think of it, I know some adults who still act this way.

These toddlers are preparing themselves for the big step forward to real "intelligence" as we usually understand it. The main indicators of intellectual development that become apparent at this age are a sense of humor, creativity, and problem-solving skills. There is a lot you can do during this time to help. In our society a high premium is put on academic achievement. If you are interested in having your child do as well as possible in school, these six months should be put to good use. It is not at all difficult; you do not have to be a college professor to furnish your child with the activities and mental stimulation he needs to make full use of his intellectual capacity. In approaching this job it is important for you to always remember not to push him too hard. Each and every child develops at a different rate and in a different way. A child learns much more rapidly if he is enjoying a particular activity. These little children also have "good" days and "bad" days, just like the rest of us. If your toddler rebels or is not interested, there is no point in trying to force him to learn or perform. As a matter of fact, if you push too hard you will not only turn him off but may even set him back.

Delayed language developments may be an early sign of autism (for example, a twelve-month-old who doesn't babble or a sixteen-month-old who doesn't say a single word). Another early clue that raises suspicion of autism is a baby who doesn't point by one year. If you notice any of these delays, your child's doctor should be consulted.

The following are the activities, toys, and equipment that I believe will be most useful in helping your child fully develop his mental capabilities:

BOOKS

As discussed earlier, the sooner you expose your baby to books, the better. All educators agree that early involvement with and love of books are among the main determining factors of future excellence in school. Growing up with books and developing a love of books will give your child a huge advantage toward achieving maximum intellectual growth.

It is sad but true that television now often takes the place of books. Sitting your little child down in front of the T.V. takes less of your time than sitting down to read a book together, but he will learn very little from T.V., especially at this age. About one-half of twelve-month-olds watch at least one hour of T.V. each day, and this is unacceptable. I advise you to follow the American Academy of Pediatrics recommendation of no T.V. at this age.

There is a wonderful organization called Reach Out and Read (www.reachoutandread.org) that supplies books to hospitals and pediatric clinics across the United States. These children's books are age-appropriate, from six months to five years, and distributed free of charge to parents to read to their children at home. Many of these children are from disadvantaged low socioeconomic families. The goal of Reach Out and Read is to help children develop literary competence and intelligence, the key to academic success. I congratulate Reach Out and Read for their efforts.

Scrapbook. I am referring to your baby's own book. All you need is some thick material such as cardboard to use for pages and some pictures of familiar objects. Work together with your toddler and paste these pictures onto the pages one by one. As you do it, talk to him about the meaning and characteristics of each picture. If he sometimes prefers to tear out the pages instead of pasting them in, so be it. He will be ready for pasting the next day or the next week or the next month. I recall a mother of a sixteen-month-old telling me that Joey's greatest pleasure was chewing up his scrapbook. My answer was, "He's pretty young to already be eating his words." I thought what I said was pretty funny, but this mother didn't even smile.

Picture books. There are many excellent picture books that you can purchase. Dr. Seuss's *Cat in the Hat* dictionary is a favorite. With your child sitting on your lap, point to a picture and say the word. He may be able to repeat the word or he may not. After awhile, when real understanding sets in, you can ask him to find the cat or the dog, and so on. Finally, if he is a verbal type, you will be able to point to a particular picture and he will say the word. This is an easy way to build up his vocabulary. Don't be discouraged if he does not actually articulate the word; this is not a sign of impaired intelligence.

Mrs. A. could not believe that her eighteen-month-old had yet to utter his first word. "What is the matter with him? He probably is not too bright," she said. On the contrary, Billy was very intelligent. He was able to point to just about everything he wanted and could understand a great many words and phrases. For example, when Billy was asked to turn on the T.V. set, he would walk right over and not only turn it on but also change the channels. Incidentally, this little fellow finally started to talk when he was about two years of age, and as his mother told me later, "It's amazing. Billy started talking practically in sentences!"

Reading. Read aloud – Mother Goose rhymes, animal stories, and the like. An ideal time for this is bedtime. Sharing a book with your baby sitting on your lap is a wonderful way to end each of his days. You will know soon enough if he is happy with your choice of book. I encourage you to make this a bedtime ritual. It is something he can always look forward to. These reading sessions are of enormous benefit and will allow him to absorb much knowledge and information.

Conversation. In a recent book, Meaningful *Differences in the Every Experience of Young Children,* Hart and Risley concluded that conversation and parent interaction through play, together with the amount of encouragement the child receives by age three, is most meaningful in affecting readiness for school and later school performance.

CRAYONS

Supply your child with a batch of different-colored crayons and give him plenty of paper. The floor is probably the best place for this activity. His art will be more impressionistic than traditional, but these crayons give him a chance to develop skill and dexterity. Working with crayons will better prepare him to master the use of a pencil and pen later on.

LANGUAGE

Language is critical for both cognitive and emotional development. Verbal competence lays the foundation for later success in school. The best way to handle language is to teach your child new words that are related to his experiences. For example, if he cuts his finger and cries, tell him that the cut hurts or that he has a "boo-boo." Talk to him about what he sees, noting not only the name of the object but its size, shape, taste, and color. Speak out loud to him about what you are doing or seeing. Point to the particular object and name it. Parallel talk is an effective method of teaching language. By this I mean talking to your child about what is happening to him at the time; for example, "Joseph is eating his cereal."

Besides talking, listen together with him to what is going on, both inside and outside the house. For example, if you both hear the telephone ring, tell him that the telephone is ringing. If you both hear thunder, talk to him about the thunder. Also take the time to listen to his responses to what you say — many parents don't wait for an answer. If he responds appropriately, be sure to show him how proud you are of his accomplishment.

Action rhymes and songs are very useful. With your toddler's increasing understanding of words and phrases, rhymes and songs are an excellent way not only to have fun together but to teach him language and concepts. I am sure that you are familiar with many of these. Two old-time favorites are "London Bridge is Falling Down" and "Ring Around the Rosie."

Passive or receptive language predominates in this period of your child's life. Passive language means that he understands what is said to him. Active language or actual talking usually is only a small part of his total language development before eighteen months of age, but the more you talk to him the sooner he will start talking back to you.

TOYS AND GAMES

Fit-together puzzles. Use only simple puzzles having no more than three pieces. These are useful for your child's hand-eye coordination and also help him learn to see and understand the concept of different shapes. You can make up your own fit-together puzzle by pasting a large picture on a piece of cardboard and then cutting it up into two or three pieces. Show him how to put the pieces together and then let him try. Don't be discouraged if he fails. Repeat the process, and sooner or later he will succeed. At that point he deserves a big kiss.

Tower building. Wooden or plastic blocks are best for this activity. Aside from the manual dexterity your toddler will develop, these blocks will teach him to manipulate variables. As he tries to build with the blocks, he learn about different sizes and shapes and sometimes even different colors. This is a problem-solving activity and so can help to prepare him to handle school problems later on, especially in understanding mathematics. What he probably will like most is knocking down the tower and starting all over again.

Sorting games. There are endless possibilities for such games all around you. For example, laundry sorting is one. With your baby nearby, sort your clean laundry into three separate piles: Mommy's, Daddy's, and the baby's. Explain to your child what each pile represents. Then mix them up and ask him to try to separate the clothes. Don't expect him to do a perfect job the first time around. Don't be surprised if your husband comes down to breakfast one morning wearing a size two toddler undershirt, or better yet, coming down wearing your sexy panties. Another example of a sorting game is taking two different sets of objects, such as a number of blocks and a number of balls, and show your baby how to separate them, the blocks on one side and balls on the other. This understanding of different groupings is basic to intelligence. For one thing, it will improve his I.Q. score on the test your toddler may take later on. Sorting and separating by group is a favorite concept used in testing intelligence.

Chores. These are splendid for learning vocabulary and word meaning. As you go about washing the dishes, ask your child to please give you a towel. Then use the towel to dry the dish. Always talk to him about what you are both doing. Putting pots away, turning off the faucets, and the like are all much more interesting than just a quiz session, which will just bore him and turn him off from learning anything.

Nesting books and staking disks. There are many to choose from and they are inexpensive. These books and disks teach your toddler to sort objects and put them in order according to size. This is useful in helping him build a foundation for mathematical thinking, and will help him when he starts school.

Follow the leader. This activity is most effective and enjoyable when played with other children. By eighteen months of age, and sometimes a bit earlier, most toddlers are ready for this. For example, tap your head, clap your hands, touch your knees, and on and on. Ask your child and his friend to do the same. This is a good learning experience and also allows your child to spend happy times with his peers.

Touching games. Simply touch an object and have your child do the same. Explain what he is feeling as he touches the object – its size, shape, texture, and color. He may not yet understand all these characteristics but he will be learning all the time. Make it a game, not a test of his knowledge.

Imitation games. For example, pull your earlobe and ask your toddler to do the same to himself. He may pull your ear instead, but after some practice, most babies at this age will begin to respond appropriately. When he does succeed, he has made a large step forward in intelligence. It will mean that his mind is starting to function on a symbolic level for the very first time. Symbolic thinking means that he can now form a picture in his mind – in this case, that he knows where his ear is without seeing it.

Water play. Since your baby probably enjoys water, it is a perfect place for him to learn. All you need are some different-sized containers. Pour water from one into the other and discuss with him what you are doing. "I am pouring the water from the little one into the big one." Then reverse the process. Next, let him try, and tell him what he is doing as he goes about pouring the water – and, of course, spilling it all over the floor.

Bath boats are also nice to have around. Let me again remind you never to leave your child alone when he is in or around water.

Animal toys. It is not enough just to give your child various animal toys. You should explain something about each one. For example, a toy duck requires a "quack-quack" to go with it and a toy cat, a "meow." Then, when you're outside with your baby and happen to see a cat, point it out to your baby and say, "That is a cat. It goes 'meow-meow.'" If that particular cat has also read this book, he will promptly "meow" himself and that will really complete this sound-effects lesson.

Cause-and-effect (If, then) games. The type of thought process involved in these games is probably the most important one of all in terms of intellectual development, and is crucial for succeeding in school. You can make these games up yourself. The purpose is to teach your child what is called relational theory: if you do this, then this will happen. Put another way, one action causes something else to happen. For example, put a toy car on a flat surface and show your baby that it does not move and that it must be pushed in order to make it go. Then put the same car on a slight incline and show him that with only a slight push, it will start rolling down the incline. Finally, put the same car on a steep incline and show him that it will roll down by itself, without being pushed. This is cause and effect or if, then. Your child also just had a lesson in momentum – and he learned about it while he was interested and having fun.

Another example of cause and effect uses various screw-top toys or simple jars. Show your child how they work. Show him how to unscrew the top. This is another if, then activity. If he does this – in this case, turns the screw top – then this will happen: the top will come off, and he can then reach into the jar.

At this age, toddlers are eager to learn and ready to take on many new challenges and tasks. Make the activities pleasurable and don't overburden your child with problems that he is either uninterested in or not yet capable of solving. Read to him, talk to him, laugh with him, and hug him. Finally, don't compare him to your neighbor's child, who may be further advanced in some of his exploits. Your baby will learn at his own rate, and if you give him the proper opportunities, he will ultimately reach his full potential.

6

Eighteen to Twenty-Four Months

"You know, Dr. Eden, I can almost see the little wheels turning in Amy's head. She is starting to think like a real person."

This mother was talking about her little twenty-month-old as I was preparing to give the baby an immunization. I might add that Amy was not only "thinking" about the needle she was about to get, but at the same time she was solving the problem she faced by running out of the examining room. Dr. Piaget refers to the eighteen- to twenty-four-month period as the "problem-solving" stage. In the mental development section of this chapter, I will discuss in some detail how babies at this age think and the tremendous advances they make in their intellectual capacities if given proper stimulation and opportunity. For purposes of introduction to this subject, the key concepts to remember are problem solving, symbolic thinking (images and ideas in the head), increased memory span, and, of course, verbal competence.

Verbal competence, both passive and active, is probably the most dramatic and obvious advance your baby will make during these marvelous and exciting six months. By age two, most babies have a speaking vocabulary of twenty words or more, and may also properly use a few two-word sentences. More important, they will learn to understand the meaning of hundreds of different words and simple phrases. As we already have stated, verbal competence is essential for your child's future academic success, and there is much that you can do to help your baby in this particular area of her development. The more talking you do to her about the world around her, the better. The more you listen to her and respond appropriately, the greater will be her chances of mastering verbal skills to her full capacity.

You will now notice that your child begins to study and investigate the quality of the objects she gets her hands on. She will feel them, drop them, chew on them, look at them, and throw them. She will be fascinated by opening and closing doors and drawers. Let her explore and practice these new skills to her heart's content. Again, try to keep your "no's" to a minimum. Make every effort not to discourage her interest and curiosity. If you fall into the trap of stopping her at every turn, you will put a damper on her zeal and drive for learning, and this will adversely affect her later school performance. I have said it before, but let me repeat it: your baby's enthusiastic search for knowledge must be encouraged in every way possible. Sleep patterns now begin to change. The total sleeping time is reduced, usually to a total of twelve hours per day. At this age, many babies try to postpone going to sleep – asking for another glass of water, another story, another kiss, etc. Don't allow this to get out of hand. Set limits, and stick to them.

It will become obvious to you that your eighteen- to twenty-four-month-old continues to be just as full of energy as before. With her increased motor skills in running and climbing, she is now more capable of exploring and experimenting. Accidents are part of growing up, especially during this time of her life, so let me again remind you to child-proof your house. Please remember that everything still goes into her mouth, so accidental poisoning is common during these six months. With your child's safety in mind, arrange her environment accordingly, then give her the space and freedom she needs in order to learn and mature. Allow her to enjoy her life to the fullest as she goes about the business of growing up.

The negative behavior patterns that no doubt have already started may well continue during this period. If you handle this aspect of your child's normal development properly, you have a better chance of looking forward to a reduction in this negative behavior by her second birthday. This reminds me of a recent incident. Mrs. B. was the proud but exhausted mother of Margaret, who not only had a mind that operated faster than her speech and emotions (which indeed is characteristic of the eighteen- to twenty-four-month-old), but also was practically a world-class example of a stubborn and negative-minded twenty-three-month-old. We had previously discussed Margaret's willfulness and temper tantrums and the fact that she was so easily frustrated. I kept reassuring Mrs. B. that much of this type of behavior would stop by the time Margaret reached two years of age. Mrs. B. and Margaret came to see me the day after her second birthday party. Nothing had changed. In fact, the birthday party was a complete disaster, with Margaret trying to confiscate all the toys from the rest of the children at the party while having a full-blown temper tantrum. All I can tell you is that Margaret is the exception; you can look forward to the fact that most children really do become less selfish, stubborn, and negative at around two years of age. I will give you my recommendations about handling negativism in the section on emotion later in this chapter.

At this time you can anticipate the start of various fears and nightmares. Actually, these fears (of thunder, lighting, dogs, and the like) are more of a problem after your child is two years old. As I have already mentioned, these eighteen- to twenty-four-month-olds are very easily frustrated; they know what they want to do but if they are not successful, they simply are not mature enough to cope. You should realize that this is all normal behavior. It is most important that you handle this properly and firmly but without becoming angry. If you don't properly sympathize with the many frustrations you baby faces, the result will be her decreased self-image and self-esteem along with the development of feelings of inferiority.

Your baby will now begin to spend more and more time in make-believe play, and you should give her the tools to do so. She will also spend more time playing by herself or enjoying the company of her friends. It is important to encourage this imaginative play. This helps her think things through and make things happen and learn in a creative way. These activities are quite important in helping to build up her self-confidence and self-reliance. In my experience, many parents are afraid to "let go." You will not be helping your child by always being around and making everything too easy for her. Now is the time in your baby's life for you to start doing some managing from the sidelines. I am not for a moment advocating that you disappear from the scene. The eighteen- to twenty-four-month-old is still both very much involved with her primary caretaker and quite dependent. The trick is to learn to strike the right balance between over-involvement and over-interference, and desertion.

Although these babies are making rapid, giant strides in developing their motor skills, verbal competence, and internal thinking and problem solving, you should be aware that they do not as yet have any concept of time (which actually does not develop much before your child is six or seven years of age). If your child is having fun, time flies; and if she is not, time drags. For example, if your child is visiting a friend and having a ball, she will not want to leave when you think it's time, not because she is mean or selfish but rather because she truly believes she has only been there for a few minutes. On the other hand, if she happens to be visiting Grandma and has been there for barely five minutes and starts to cry because she wants to leave, it is not only because she is not having a good time but also because she honestly thinks that she's already been there forever.

Let me bring up the subject of television. It is true that a few eighteen- to twenty-four-month-olds may watch some T.V. and find it interesting. But for all practical purposes it's a waste of time for most children that age, and I would discourage any television watching until your child reaches age two (the whole subject of television watching will be discussed in the next chapter). Further, I am also not a big fan of so-called educational videogames in general, but at this age I certainly would advise you not to bother with them.

Each and every day is important in your child's growth. Your child is more than ready to practice her increasing skills: motor, verbal, and mental. It's a shame if any of these are slowed down during this most important stage of her development. Keep in mind that her personality is being shaped day by day, in large measure by how she is being treated.

To sum up, I would advise that you make every effort to watch your child in action as carefully as possible and listen to her as she goes about her daily tasks. If you are properly attuned to your baby, you soon realize that she can often "tell" you, without using the actual words, exactly how she feels and what she needs. As Dr. Burton White points out in *The First Three Years of Life,* a balanced approach is what is needed at this age—and, as a matter of fact, at any age. I agree completely with him that parents who concentrate too much effort and time, for example, on verbal competence at the expense of physical development and nutrition are making a serious mistake. As you surely must have noticed by now, each chapter in this book places equal emphasis on the physical, mental, and emotional development of the child; similarly, each of these areas requires your equal attention. A relaxed approach is most effective. Laughing with your child and having fun with her is without question the best way to raise her. Too many parents take the job too seriously and seem to forget about their own as well as their child's sense of humor. Babies are funny, and at this age already have developed a fine sense of humor. If given half a chance they laugh a lot, and despite their many frustrations and anxieties, have a marvelous, happy time of it. In terms of the future, a happy child develops to her full potential much more easily than a child raised in a house without laughter.

GROWTH AND DEVELOPMENT

Physical (Motor)

18–24 MONTHS

- Walks up and down stairs.
- Runs well and usually can stop short without falling on face.
- Skillful and adventuresome climber.
- Can build towers of up to five or six blocks.
- Kicks balls.
- Throws balls, occasionally toward target.
- Usually begins to prefer one hand over the other.
- Learns to turn pages one at a time.
- Scribbles with crayon or pencil.
- Dances to music.
- Feeds herself efficiently using spoon and cup (can even handle peeling a banana).
- Does everything as fast as possible, e.g., running, eating, climbing, emptying drawers.

Note: These charts are based on average ranges of growth and development; many normal babies perform and achieve either sooner or later than indicated.

GROWTH AND DEVELOPMENT

Emotional (Social)

18-24 MONTHS

- May begin having nightmares during sleep.
- The real start of make-believe play.
- Easily frustrated.
- Stubborn; wants her own way.
- Involved in negative behavior but still enjoys pleasing others.
- Demands attention.
- Enjoys changes of environment and scenery.
- Helps with chores around the house with enthusiasm and energy.
- May develop fears, e.g., of water, dogs, thunder, or lightning.
- Displays selfish behavior; possessive of her toys and belongings.
- Behavior becomes better and better organized.
- Plays well with other children (usually around her second birthday).
- Her two favorite words are "no" and "mine."
- May start to know when bowel movement is about to happen.

Note: These charts are based on average ranges of growth and development; many normal babies perform and achieve either sooner or later than indicated.

GROWTH AND DEVELOPMENT

MENTAL (INTELLECTUAL)

18-24 MONTHS

- Learns to draw a line or circle with crayon after proper instruction.
- Understands and follows simple instruction.
- Points to appropriate picture in book when asked.
- Develops usable vocabulary of up to twenty words and a few short phrases, e.g., "Mama go bye-bye."
- Listens to and enjoys simple stories.
- Can point to and name different parts of her body.
- Tells you what she wants, with either gestures or words.
- Fits various puzzles together.
- Refers to herself by name.
- Matches similar objects and groups of objects.
- Helps undress herself.
- Spends long periods of time just observing or staring (she's "thinking").
- The start of "symbolic thinking" and "thoughtfulness."
- Problem-solving capacity increases day by day.

Note: These charts are based on average ranges of growth and development; many normal babies perform and achieve either sooner or later than indicated.

PHYSICAL (MOTOR) DEVELOPMENT

In all likelihood your baby will now be drinking cow's milk, either from a bottle or from a cup. For those mothers who are still breast-feeding, there is no reason to stop. If both you and your baby are still enjoying the breast-feeding experience, then by all means continue it. You will find that your child will usually "tell" you one way or another when she has finally had enough of breast-feeding. Each example that I have included in the book thus far is true, including the following, which you really may find hard to believe. Mrs. S. was a relaxed and loving mother who was having a marvelous time breast-feeding Carole, a delightful, happy, friendly, and, at two years of age, very verbal child. When Carole was fifteen months old I asked Mrs. S. if she planned to stop breast-feeding soon. "Absolutely not; why should I?" she answered. I certainly had no objection to her continuing to breast-feed, and for the next two well-baby visits, at eighteen months and twenty-one months of age, I did not bring up the subject. At each of these visits Mrs. S. informed me that she was still breast-feeding her daughter and that everything was fine. At the two-year-old visit the first words out of Mrs. S.'s mouth were, "Dr. Eden, I've stopped breast-feeding. Would you believe that last week right in the middle of a feeding, Carole suddenly stopped, turned her head away from the breast, made a face, and told me, 'Wan' chocolate milk.'"

As I outlined in the previous chapter, babies over one year of age no longer require large quantities of milk each day. If your child drinks anywhere from twelve to sixteen ounces of milk per day, this is sufficient for her nutritional needs, as long as, in addition, she is offered the well-balanced diet that we presented earlier. Give her a daily iron-fortified multi-vitamin preparation to continue preventing iron-deficiency. Offer her a well-balanced diet, including plenty of fruit and vegetables. Most eighteen- to twenty-four-months-olds handle a spoon and cup extremely well and usually can feed themselves without any difficulty. In addition to handling the spoon and cup, they can do even more – for example, peeling a banana. I would discourage you from getting into the habit of force-feeding your baby when and if she doesn't clean her plate. I would also advise you not to coax, cajole, threaten, or offer her a reward to get her to complete her meal. I have mentioned this before but let me repeat it: allow you child to end the meal when she thinks it's over rather than when you think she has eaten enough.

I am often asked about the amounts of various foods a child should eat. There is no specific answer to that question. Each and every baby has different requirements, a different appetite, and a different point of satiation. What I can tell you is that I have rarely seen a mother under feed her baby. Rather, the opposite is usually the case. A little child does not need as many calories as an adult, and the child's portions of food should be smaller than your own. I must admit that there are exceptions. A certain percentage of babies have voracious appetites and they eat just about anything and everything you put in front of them. We will be discussing this subject and the whole subject of establishing proper eating patterns in the next chapter (Two to Three Years). One point that I would like to make now is that it is a good idea to offer your child relatively small portions at each meal. If she is still hungry after finishing, she will tell you, and you can then replenish her plate. This is a much more sensible approach than loading up her dish with huge quantities of food that she surely should not and cannot finish. This one simple piece of advice will go a long way in starting to instill proper eating habits. If you start this now, the chances are better that these habits will remain with her as she grows up and will help lower the risk of her becoming obese.

We have already discussed how babies develop tastes for certain foods. They learn to like what you offer them; it is really as simple as that. If you offer your baby plenty of fruits, vegetables, yogurt, and the like, she will continue to enjoy these nutritious foods as she grows older. On the other hand, if you start giving her a steady diet of soda, cookies, and candy, she will grow up craving this type of junk food and will continue to eat that way all her life. Don't be afraid to offer a variety of different nutritious foods. That is the only way she will learn to eat and enjoy the well-balanced diet that is so important for her future well-being.

My advice is not to allow yourself to fall into the trap of appeasing and bribing your child with junk foods. Snacking between meals is fine, but it depends on what kind of snacks you use. Unfortunately, the usual between-meal foods are low in nutritive value and too high in calories, saturated fat, and refined sugar (more about this when we take up the subject of television in the next chapter). Typical unworthy snacks include soft drinks, potato chips, cookies, and candy bars. Some excellent snacks that should always be available for your baby are plain yogurt, carrots, pieces of apple, and natural fruit juice. Please take my word for it: if you consistently offer your child this type of snack between meals instead of junk food, she will quickly learn to love and ask for them. I would also avoid excessively salty snacks, such as salted peanuts and pretzels. In terms of her future physical health, developing correct eating patterns now is essential.

You must continue to remain on the alert for obesity. If your baby looks fat, call it to her doctor's attention. It is less likely that she will become too fat if you are careful in terms of the size of the portions and the selection of the between-meal snacks you offer her. An incredible statistic is that, in the United Stated, between twenty and forty percent of all the calories eaten each day are consumed in the form of between-meal snacks. It is a fact that a fat child is not a healthy child, at any age.

I would like to call to your attention to a very recent large-scale investigation of more than 1,000 healthy children that was carried out by the

United States National Institute of Child Health and Human Development Early Child Care Research Network. The results demonstrated that overweight two- and three-year-olds were over five times more likely to be overweight at age twelve than normal weight two- and three-year-olds. The time to start preventing obesity is now.

In the next chapter, I will discuss the so-called prudent type of diet that is recommended for all children over two years of age. For now, I would encourage you to continue to keep the number of eggs you feed your baby down to three to four per week and continue to cut down on added salt and sugar. Offer you baby chicken, veal, and fish more often than red and fatty meats such as pork and beef.

To close this section on nutrition, I'd like to remind you that mealtimes can and should be fun. Try very hard to make your child's mealtimes happy experiences. This is easier said than done, but it is important to make the attempt. Be relaxed and cheerful as you offer your youngster a well-balanced, variety-filled, and nutritious diet. In such an environment your child will begin to associate this healthy diet with good feelings all around. Such a pleasant eating environment is more conducive for your child to continue to eat the same foods as she grows up. It is much easier to establish proper eating patterns early in life then to try to modify them later on.

EXERCISE

Your child's normal energy levels are such that there is very little you need to do to ensure that she exercises sufficiently. If we could only figure out a way to harness all this energy, we would put the OPEC countries out of business (especially important with the current price of gasoline). Eighteen- to twenty-four-month-olds run and jump and climb and have excellent muscle coordination. Your child will learn to kick and throw a ball and will maneuver up and down the stairs without difficulty. If you do not put insurmountable roadblocks in her way because you are afraid of accidents, she will take care of most of her exercise requirements all by herself.

Before listing my specific recommendations for physical activities during this period, I want to caution you against using your television set as a method for keeping your child quiet and in one place. Many parents unconsciously encourage the start of a sedentary lifestyle in their children by sitting them down in front of the T.V. set, usually armed with cookies and candy. I suggested earlier that most eighteen- to twenty-four-month-olds do not appreciate or learn very much from T.V., but if your child's dish is continuously replenished with goodies as she sits in front of the set, she will in short order learn to enjoy this time-wasting inactivity. This can be the start of a vicious cycle resulting in a child becoming too fat and flabby and losing all desire to be active. In one of my previous books about childhood obesity the title of one of the chapters was "The S.O.B. Syndrome." No, it didn't stand for the usual meaning of S.O.B. Rather, it referred to "The Sitting on Butt Syndrome." It can start at this young age, so beware.

SPECIFIC RECOMMENDATIONS

The specific suggestions that I believe will insure that your child develops to her maximum physical capacity are by and large the same activities listed in the previous chapter. There are some changes in emphasis and degree of sophistication. Except for a four-wheeled vehicle of one kind or another, little additional equipment need be purchased during these six months.

Push- and pull-toys. These are still very enjoyable; in fact, they are probably more fun now, as your child really is involved in make-believe play, is more coordinated, and has more skill in handling them.

Balls. The games that you can play with your child at this age are more advanced and sophisticated than before. One activity that I remember enjoying with each of my children was sitting on the floor with our feet touching and rolling a large, light ball back and forth. As we pushed the ball back and forth, I talked about what we were doing: "Robert, your turn. Good. Now Daddy's turn." These ball games advanced from rolling to throwing the ball, and finally, to learning how to catch it. My daughter, Liz, enjoyed kicking the ball most and so we improvised a soccer type of game on the rug (after putting away anything breakable).

Games involving balls of various sizes and shapes can be played with more than one child at a time and can be a source of great pleasure for your child and her friends. Her coordination, muscle tone, strength, and agility all are helped by such activities. This is very important for her future, not only in terms of improved physical health and vigor but also in terms of improved self-image and self-confidence. Physical exercises and the acquisition of physical skills help to develop a positive body image (this subject will be discussed more fully in the next chapter).

Crawling games. Although your child is now standing and walking and running more and more of the time, she still enjoys crawling around. Encourage her to do so with various rug games.

Pounding bench. There are a number of these on the market. They usually include a hammer and large pegs and a bench. Hammering the pegs into the bench is fine for hand-eye coordination and also serves to increase muscle strength. When your child learns to hammer the pegs in efficiently, she will feel very proud of herself, and you should tell her how proud you are of her accomplishment.

Roughhouse activities. Continue your roughhouse activities – and don't leave out the girls.

MYTH: Little girls are more fragile and delicate, and weaker than little boys.

An eighteen- to twenty-four-month-old girl is just as strong, sturdy, and active as a boy of that age. I recall a twenty-month-old little girl whose greatest pleasure in life was wrestling with her older brother and her father. Mr. T. called me up one day to ask me about this. "Is this kind of rough exercise good for Cathy?" My answer was an emphatic "Yes." Both boys and girls should be encouraged in every way possible to participate in vigorous and rigorous physical activity. Starting such activity at this very young age does much to ensure that they will continue on the road to a lifestyle that includes taking proper care of and developing pride in their bodies.

Outdoor play or park. This was discussed in the previous chapter. Obviously it is very important that your child continue to engage in these outdoor activities. I would just add that if you have not yet purchased some type of climbing equipment for your child, this would be a good time to do so. The eighteen- to twenty-four-month-old is fascinated by climbing and is becoming more and more skillful at it.

Four-wheeled vehicle. A number of styles are available. Your child can sit on or straddle the vehicle and maneuver herself around on it. This is great exercise, and also serves to prepare your child for her first tricycle. Very few children are really ready for a tricycle much before two years of age, so I would advise you not buy one yet.

Chores. In the previous chapter, chores were discussed in the section on mental development. I am including chores in the physical development section of this chapter for a specific reason. An eighteen- to twenty-four-month-old is quite strong and willing and able to work. Therefore, it is good practice to get your child involved now in helping around the house. This will help her physical development and help to instill a sense of cooperation in her. I am referring to carrying out the garbage, moving small pieces of furniture, carrying packages, and running to call another member of the family to the phone. All these chores are well within her physical capabilities. They are all good exercise and useful as well. If you think about it, there is nothing a preschool or schoolteacher appreciates more than a child willing and able to cooperate and help in the classroom. Keep this fact in mind as you involve your youngster with various household chores.

There is an old wives' tale that I want to repeat a second time to complete this section:

MYTH: Cold air is unhealthy for little children and can cause respiratory infections and even pneumonia.

There is no truth to this one. The fact is that respiratory infections of all kinds are caused by a virus or bacteria and are not related to cold weather. I have included this myth here again to encourage you to take your child outside every chance you get, including cold days. It is unfair to coop up an active young child during the winter months. The more opportunities she has to run and jump and climb, the stronger and healthier she will become.

SAFETY TIPS

Choking. All your baby's toys should be unbreakable and have no small parts or sharp edges. Keep your child away from chewing gum, popcorn, peanuts, and small balls. It is easy for a baby to choke.

Burns and electric shocks. Never leave your child unattended in the kitchen; it is a danger area. Teach her the meaning of hot. Always keep matches out of sight. While cooking, get into the habit of only using the back burners and turning the pot handles to the wall. As part of your child-proofing, cover your electrical outlets with safety plugs if you have not already done so. Place guards in front of wall heaters, fireplaces, and steam radiators. Be especially careful with electrical cords that are attached to coffee pots and the like. This is a common cause of severe burns.

Poisons. Since everything goes into her mouth, poisoning is quite common during this period. It is important to realize that babies do not seem to worry about the odors of various substances. The smell, no matter how unpleasant it might be to you, does not act as a deterrent to a child. Here are some suggestions about dealing with poisonous substances in your home:

1. Always keep products in their original containers. Never put inedible products into food or beverage containers.
2. Always read the label carefully before using any product.
3. Since your child is a great imitator, get into the habit of not taking any medicine when she is around.

4. Get rid of any oil of wintergreen you might have in the house. This is a deadly poison with no therapeutic value.

We had a recent case of oil of wintergreen poisoning at the hospital with which I am affiliated. A two-year-old drank one teaspoon of it. That small amount can be a lethal dose of salicylates, and we were fortunate that the baby survived.

5. Statistics have shown that children who have ingested a poisonous substance one time are more likely to do it again. Therefore, if your child already has been involved with a poison, be especially alert and careful so that it will not happen again.

6. It is gratifying to report that the death rates from poisoning in the United States in the past ten years have decreased along with the appearance of regulated safety packaging on containers of aspirin, furniture polish, drain cleaners, prescriptions, and the like. Nevertheless, many children under the age of two still die each year of accidental poisoning.

Guns. It is best to keep all firearms out of the house if at all possible. Studies show that children in homes with guns are in more danger of shooting themselves or friends accidentally than being hurt by an intruder. Handguns are especially dangerous.

Drowning. Again, never leave your child alone in or near a bathtub or wading or swimming pool, even for a second. A baby can drown in less than two inches of water.

EMOTIONAL (SOCIAL) DEVELOPMENT

The question of toilet training is often raised at around this age. I have chosen to discuss it in the next chapter (Two to Three Years) because I believe that any serious attempts at training your child should not start much before the age of two. It is true, however, that some eighteen- to twenty-four-month-olds are ready to be toilet trained. If you think that this may be the case with your child, read about my approach in the next chapter.

There are three important general areas related to the emotional development of your child that I want to discuss with you before giving you specific recommendations for helping her achieve maximum emotional maturity: discipline, slowing down, and body talk.

DISCIPLINE

Negative behavior and temper tantrums should be expected, and there is no sense in kidding you – they can be very difficult to manage. Some call this period of your child's life an early form, or better yet, a preview, of her adolescent rebellion period later on.

All of us surely agree that children must be taught to control their behavior on a day-to-day basis so that they can eventually learn to rely on themselves, rather than on adults, to decide what is right and what is wrong. However, there are large areas of disagreement in terms of how best to accomplish this. The word discipline comes from the word "disciple," meaning someone who follows the teaching of another. Discipline therefore refers to the learning experiences you give your child, and does not simply mean punishment. I recently asked ten consecutive mothers of eighteen- to twenty-four-month-olds during their office visits to give me their definition of discipline. Seven out of the ten said punishment. Only three talked about teaching and learning. The word discipline is derived from disciple, meaning pupil – please remember this. Unfortunately, many parents as well as professionals equate discipline with punishment. Discipline does not mean punishment, it means teaching. When a child misbehaves, she often does so to show her independence, learn a new skill (such as smashing dishes on the floor), or express her feeling of frustration. From her point of view these are all sound and valid reasons for her negative behavior. I am not for a moment advocating that you should always approve of what she does. There will be times when you will have to act promptly in order to stop her from hurting herself or somebody else. But at least if you understand why she is acting up in this fashion, you will be in a better position to cope with it.

Frustrated and angry parents sometimes react by striking out at their misbehaving child, either physically or verbally. I believed that this not only is the wrong way to teach your child anything, but it doesn't work. Instilling fear in your child is not the way to teach her right from wrong.

Some examples of poor discipline techniques are the following:

Corporal punishment. Shaming, humiliating, or beating a child all are psychologically damaging and, as far as I am concerned, examples of child abuse, and besides, they don't work. Abuse and fear of abuse are terrible ways to motivate your child and will surely impair her social skills and development as well as her own parenting skills. The fact is that abused children often become child abusers as adults.

Screaming and yelling. Sometimes you just can't control yourself, but it gets you nowhere, increasing the conflict and provoking more disruptive behavior. Remember, children learn by example.

Labeling. If you call your child "bad" often enough she will start believing you, and that certainly will not help her self-image and self-worth. When she misbehaves she is not bad, she just hasn't yet learned to behave properly. Your job is to teach her, not call her derogatory names.

There are a number of proper techniques that can help teach your child to change her behavior, stop her destructive tendencies and temper tantrums, and encourage self-control and self-discipline. Here are some:

Distract her. This may not work too well at this age, but it is worth a try. Whenever possible, try to distract or redirect your child to another activity. For example, try playing some music or sing a song together. As the old saying goes, "Music has charms to soothe a savage beast," and sometimes it also soothes a savage child.

Separation. One effective method of disciplining (teaching) your child when she misbehaves is to simply take her away from the place of trouble. For example, if she is in the park playing and suddenly decides to bite her friend, separate her from the situation and take her back home.

Explanation. If you find it necessary to remove your child from an area or activity because of her misbehavior, try to explain to her why you are doing so. Establishing a rule or regulation and not explaining why you have done so will make it very difficult for your child to understand and adhere to the rules. Set the rules clearly.

Compromise. You and your child will have many, many differences of opinion, and every once in a while it is helpful if you give in and let your child have her way. Babies learn from their mistakes and so whenever possible, ignore the misbehavior or at least forgive her. If you are having a dispute whose outcome is not particularly important, that is the time to compromise. To put it another way, allow your child to make some decisions on her own. Let her win some of the small arguments and you'll have a better chance of winning the big ones. No biting is one of the big ones. There are no compromises here.

Punishment. There is a place for punishment in teaching discipline. Always explain to your child the consequences of her behavior ahead of time. When punishment is used it should always teach a lesson. Sending her to bed for not putting her toys away teaches her nothing. But rather, not allowing her to play with those toys for a while will help her understand the situation. Spanking your child should be reserved only for very important situations. Some examples of what I call very important situations include a child who decides to turn on the gas jets on the stove or runs out into the street. The appropriate punishment for less important situations is to take away certain privileges. If you punish her too often for every minor infraction of the rules, any type of punishment, including spanking, will lose its effectiveness.

Since West Point does not accept one-and-a-half or even two year olds, I advise you not to treat your child as though she were in military school. There are times when you will have to put your foot down and take firm action. Save those occasions for the moments that really count, and look the other way when her misbehavior is merely a little out of line.

SLOWING DOWN

This is a subject that very few parents think about. If you find that you always seem to be in a hurry because you are so very busy, your little child may be getting the wrong message from you. She cannot yet understand that you really have so much to do each day. She will start to think that she is just not important enough for you to spend much time with her. I realize that sometimes there just are not enough hours in the day to get everything done, but nonetheless you should try to slow down and spend more time holding and touching and talking to your child. Bathing, feeding, and dressing her on the run is not enough. Your child must be reassured of your love every single day, and this takes a certain amount of quiet time besides lots of good intentions. If you can't find at least one half-hour each day for your baby, there is something drastically wrong with your schedule and I suggest you do something about it.

BODY TALK

Despite the fact that your child's usable vocabulary is growing during these six months, your baby will still do a lot of her "talking" with her body and through her behavior. Many of us do not pay enough attention to this body language because we assume that at this age, the child will communicate her needs to us verbally. Actually, without using any recognizable words, your child still can give you many clues as to what she wants – by her expression, gestures, tone of voice, various moods, and actions. You can rest assured that she will get your attention one way or another. If you are not attuned to what she wants, she may smash her favorite toy in frustration or have a full-blown temper tantrum. The point I am trying to make is that you should "listen" to your child's body talk and respond appropriately. If she is unable to make her wishes known to you over and over again because she does not yet have the verbal competence to do so and you cannot understand her body language, she may become discouraged, withdrawn, negative, or hostile.

SPECIFIC RECOMMENDATIONS

The following are my specific recommendations for helping your child's emotional development:

Make-believe games. During these six months, many babies start make-believe play, although some don't do very much of this until after their second birthday. Your child will now develop a better sense of reality and real sense of "self." Because of this, imaginative play is very useful in helping her deal with her feelings. For example, she will now be able to scold or yell at her doll or, if she feels like it, kiss and cuddle the doll instead. She can play "mama" and she has a vehicle through which to express her feelings. Psychologists call this role playing. Of course, now she can also talk to her doll. Most of the time you won't be able to understand what she is saying but as long as the doll understands, everything is fine. For these make-believe games, supply your child with a variety of dolls and stuffed animals. Also give her a toy telephone, which is not only a great prop for make-believe conversations, but also helps build up her language skills. Dump trucks, toy carriages, and toy fire engines are very much appreciated by all young children, along with empty boxes of all shapes and sizes.

It should be easy for you to improvise all sorts of make-believe games, and I can assure you that your child will enjoy all of them. For example, take one of her crayons and teach her to imagine that it is not a crayon but a car. After awhile she will understand what you are doing and join the fun. She may take another crayon and use it as a car herself or she may go to her toy chest and bring out a real toy car instead.

By giving her the tools to deal more easily with her own feelings, you will help to build up her emotional stability and feelings of self-worth, and these feeling will remain with her as she grows and matures.

At about this age, nightmares may begin. With the start of symbolic-level thinking (to be discussed in the section on mental development), nightmares occur. This is an example of distorted reality. I have been called many times by parents and told about nightmares occurring soon after one traumatic experience or another. I was even blamed for one little boy's nightmare because it took place the very night after I had sutured a laceration on his head that was associated with much screaming and yelling.

Chores. Although I discussed chores in the physical development section of this chapter, I am including them here too because household chores are an effective way to teach your child about cooperation, and they also help to make her feel that she is a real part of the family. The sooner she learns about cooperation and being part of the family, the better.

Promises and threats. With negativism, stubbornness, and selfishness all integral parts of your child's behavior at this age, it will be very easy for you to make idle threats or promises that you will not be able or want to keep. I remember one mother who was so upset with her twenty-month-old son's behavior that she threatened never to let Michael visit his friends if he did not immediately stop tearing up his books. Never is a little too long. My advice is never make a promise or a threat unless you are prepared to stick to your word.

A study sponsored by the National Institute of Mental Health concluded that parents who kept their promises had children who grew up to be trusting parents. Parents who are careless about or unable to keep their promises or promise their children anything to keep them quiet or change their behavior do irreparable harm. These parents cause their children to develop deep suspicions of others and a pessimistic approach to life.

Music. Most eighteen- to twenty-four-month-olds can learn to use a push-in type of record player after they've been given a few demonstrations. Such a record player will allow your child to decide for herself when to play music. Little children should be encouraged to dance and move rhythmically in time to music since this is a splendid way for them to learn to become more attuned to their bodies. In the next chapter (Two to Three Years), I will be discussing the concept of positive body image and what you can do to help your child learn to love her own body. For now, let me say that learning to dance is one way of helping to achieve a good feeling about one's own body. Playing rhythm instruments (as mentioned in the previous chapter) remains a fine activity for your child. A house that is full of music (even if the music may not exactly be to your own taste) is a happier place for your child.

Play-doh. This is helpful for creative and dramatic play. Play-doh is less messy than regular clay and is reusable if it is kept in a closed, airtight container when not in use. Some parents complain about the way it smells, but children don't seem to mind the odor. Your child can mold it into various shapes and forms and will take great pride in her artwork.

"Let-go" time. Your little child now requires more time for herself. She will be initiating her own activities and playing on her own, and you should encourage her. By allowing her this independence, you will be preparing her to face future activities outside the home, such as at a day care center or nursery school. We call the time your child spends by herself "let-go" time. It is hard for some parents to believe or accept the fact that their children simply don't need them all the time. Your eighteen- to twenty-four-month-old must be given the opportunity to fend for herself part of each day, so don't be afraid to let go.

An example of let-go time is when you are home doing your chores in one room or area of the house while your baby is playing by herself in another room. Every once in a while she will come to you to make sure that you are still around and perhaps to show you what she is doing, and then she will go back to her own activity. This is fine for her independence and feeling of self-worth. Such an arrangement helps her become her own person. It is important that you (or the primary caretaker) be where she can find you. If you let go too fast or too far – such as, for example, suddenly disappearing entirely from the scene without telling her – your child will become very frightened and insecure. If you do this too often, chances are she will start hanging onto your apron strings all day long because she will always be afraid that you will desert her again.

Self-esteem. Because I have repeated it so often, you probably are getting the idea that I believe very strongly that building up your child's self-esteem and self-image is one of the most important contributions you can ever make to her future emotional well-being and success in school and beyond. You are right, that is exactly what I believe. Helping to give your little child a positive sense of self-worth is truly one of the major commandments of being a positive parent. If you continuously "put her down," criticize, and correct her, and make her feel inadequate and stupid (however well-intentioned your motives may be), you will cause her to become unsure of herself and less confident in her own abilities. This will result in her losing interest and initiative in learning, simply because she will be afraid of failing again. She will stop trying as hard. This will be reflected in her later school and work performance. Always encourage rather than discourage your child. Neither expect nor demand perfection. Setting unrealistic goals is the surest and fastest way to destroy your child's self-confidence.

Curiosity. Continue to encourage your child's curiosity and adventurous spirit. If she happens to fail in a task, don't reprimand her. Rather, tell her that it is perfectly all right. Show her that you're happy she tried, and don't worry about whether or not she is successful. It is only by trying that she will eventually learn, and if she is secure in the knowledge that you are not judging her each time, she will remain enthusiastic and anxious to expand her learning experiences. Chances are that how she thinks about herself now will probably be how she thinks of herself later on, when she starts school. With her curiosity and optimism intact, she is much more likely to be successful.

To end this section, I would like to get rid of another old wives' tale:

MYTH: Thumb sucking at this age is a sure sign of emotional trouble.
Not true at all. The majority of children who are still sucking their thumbs between eighteen and twenty-four months of age are not at all emotionally

disturbed. They just enjoy sucking their thumbs. I might add that there is another myth about thumb sucking – that it will ruin the child's permanent teeth alignment. Again, not true. It is true that with vigorous thumb sucking the baby teeth may be pushed out of line, but if the thumb sucking stops before age four, it is very unlikely that the permanent teeth will be affected.

MENTAL (INTELLECTUAL) DEVELOPMENT

I want to start this section with a warning: Don't try to push your little child too hard or too fast. With her remarkable advances in real thinking, it will be very easy for you to inadvertently overburden her learning capacity during these six months. Too much stimulation has been shown to be just as detrimental to optimum mental development as too little stimulation. It has been shown that too much practice will make a child's response so automatic that an appropriate response will be more difficult to elicit when she is faced with a new learning situation. For example, if your child is given the same puzzle to solve over and over again and then finally is presented with a new puzzle, she will automatically respond to it in the same way she responded to the old one. This is called stereotyping, and it can result in developmental delays at any stage of concept development.

Another danger of overburdening is related to an over-enriched environment, one that offers your child more than she can cope with. Children enjoy problem solving, but problems that are beyond their capabilities turn them off completely. If a child is faced with many problems that she is not ready and able to solve, she will withdraw and retreat and lose interest in solving any problems. What I mean is that it is just as bad to expect too much from your child as it is to not challenge her mind at all. The trick is to try to make sure that what you offer her neither bores nor frustrates her but rather provides her with the environment that will stimulate her so that she can develop her intellectual capacities and competencies to their fullest.

Your child's mind now starts to function on a symbolic level. Your child is capable of storing and remembering images and ideas in her brain. An excellent example that explains symbolic thinking is presented in *Help Your Baby Learn,* by Stephen Lehane. He describes the eighteen-month-old daughter of two blind parents who was trying to avoid being found by her father. This child wore bells on her shoes so that her blind parents could more easily locate where she was. This girl was observed to shuffle along slowly and gingerly step backward because she realized that this type of movement would silence the ringing of the bells. She understood that she was actually fooling her father and held her hands up to her face, trying to control her giggling and laughing because she also understood that her noises would have betrayed her location. At one-and-a-half years of age she not only had figured out the principle of not making noise with the bells and with her laughter, but she also was already able to manipulate and fool her parents. This very young lady was able to solve a most complicated and complex problem.

Your child will now begin to understand the concept of alternatives and options. This is that start of real thinking ability, of "thoughtfulness." She will be able to understand explanations and will have a pretty clear understanding of reality. What all this means is that the eighteen- to twenty-four-month-old starts figuring thing out all by herself, which is a remarkable and exciting advance in her mental competency. Her problem-solving ability becomes more sophisticated. For example, she learns to use a stick to push a ball off a high shelf when she can't reach it with her hands. Abstract thinking also becomes part of her intellectual armamentarium. Whereas previously she understood that her block was the only block there was, now she learns the concept of a block. In other words, she now realizes that there are all sorts of different-sized, different-shaped, and different-colored blocks with one common denominator: the characteristics of a block. This holds true for bottles, dishes, balls, and other objects.

The eighteen- to twenty-four-month-old also usually learns to master an additional and difficult concept called conservation, a sign of intelligence as we know it.

CONSERVATION

The concept of conservation means that a child understands that an object is the same even though it actually looks different when its shape is changed. It also means that she realizes that the weight of an object is unrelated to any change in its shape. Before this, a child believes that all objects are the same weight, and that the larger or longer the object, the heavier it is. When you think about it, the ability to make this transition in perception is indeed a remarkable advance in a child's intellectual ability.

VERBAL COMPETENCE

As I mentioned at the beginning of this chapter, you will now see great strides forward in verbal competence. By age two, your child probably will have a working vocabulary of twenty words or more and also will be able to say a few simple two-word phrases. She will start to ask for things with words and may start using the word "me." Instead of using her own name she will begin to say "me want." Although the results are in a sense obvious, you might be interested in an anthropological study conducted at Stanford University by Dr. Chevalier-Skolnikoff that involved infant apes and infant humans during the first two years of life. The results demonstrated an almost identical behavior pattern month by month in both groups, with one essential difference: The infant apes' vocalization process stopped at an early age, and this is considered the vital factor in the subsequent maturation of both species. Apes never coo or babble and never acquire more sophisticated modes of vocalization. The important point to remember is that speech and language appear to be the principal mode of future learning and socialization. Put another way, language is what separates humans from the rest of the animal kingdom. Helping your child acquire verbal competence is most important for her future intellectual accomplishments.

Before giving you my specific recommendations to help your child reach her maximum intellectual potential, allow me to put to rest another widely held misconception that relates to mental development.

MYTH: A fever convulsion causes brain damage.

Not true. The type of convulsion that is caused only by high fever (most occur between six months and two years) does not result in brain damage. Such a seizure can be very frightening, but if handled properly, is easily managed. Discuss this subject with your child's physician so that you know what to do if and when it happens.

SPECIFIC RECOMMENDATIONS

Below are some specific recommendations about activities and equipment (your child will invent many other activities on her own, and should be encouraged to do so).

Puzzles. The more, the merrier. Your child is getting better at solving puzzles all the time. She will learn to put together simple jigsaw puzzles. You can make your own with construction paper or cardboard. All you have to do is cut out various shapes and show her what to do. This type of puzzle will help her learn about size, position, and shape. You can also buy wooden or plastic puzzles, always making sure they are simple, with just a few familiar objects. Modular sets to fit together are also useful for building and learning about design and increasing her manual dexterity.

Guessing games. Among these, a favorite is a takeoff on the well-known "shell game" used by gamblers to fleece unsuspecting and greedy participants. All you need are three different-sized cans and a toy small enough to fit under each of the cans. Place the toy under one of them and show your baby what you have done. Next, move the cans around and then ask her to tell you where the toy is. If she guesses right, you both should be very happy. If she makes a mistake, don't get upset, but say, "No, it is not there. Try again." In a relatively short period of time she should be able to get the hang of it, and then it's time to move on to a more difficult version. This time, actually hide the toy under one of the cans, always remembering to hide it under the largest one, and ask her to find it. It will take varying amounts of time, but sooner or later she will realize what you are doing and will be able to pick out the correct (largest) can. If you stop to think about it, this is quite an accomplishment. She has been able to reason and figure out that the toy is always hidden under the largest can. Another variation is to turn things around and ask her to hide the toy and have you guess. Colored cans or cans with different labels can be used as well. Remember always to hide the toy in a consistent manner so that the game does not become strictly one of guessing.

Never make things too difficult for your child, and above all, don't tease or criticize her when she makes a mistake. There are endless variations you can devise. This kind of activity teaches your child about space relations, size, shape, and location, and promotes reasoning and problem-solving ability. It is so effective because it is challenging, lots of fun, and never boring.

Going places. I have said it before and I will say it again: it is important to take your child out of the house as often as possible – to the park, zoo, museum, and airport. Trips in the automobile, to children's theaters, and to restaurants should be planned whenever possible. Your child will enjoy these expeditions and will have the opportunity to absorb much valuable information, provided you take the time to talk to her and explain exactly what she is seeing and doing. Since children at this age understand up to several hundred different words and phrases, they are more than ready to listen and respond to what you have to say.

Anatomy. It is quite important for your child to learn about the various parts of her body and their functions. Little children are fascinated with their bodies and are anxious to learn all they can. Point and ask, "Where is your mouth? Your vagina?" I am amazed by how many different strange words parents use to identify that part of their little girls' anatomy instead of vagina. "Where are your eyes?" Teach her what each part of her body does. For example, ears are for hearing, eyes for seeing, and mouths for opening and chewing. Cover your child's eyes and then say, "Now you can't see." I once was witness to an amazing show of knowledge in anatomy put on by a mother and her twenty-one-month-old girl. That child not only knew the obvious parts of her body but also could point, without making a single mistake, to her clavicle, sternum, knee, wrist, and as a matter of fact, to just about every single part of her little body. I did not ask, but I am pretty sure that Mrs. P. was preparing her daughter for early entry into medical school!

Functions of objects. There is no reason to dwell on this in great detail. It is obvious that teaching your child the functions of the various objects she sees is the cornerstone of her learning process. If you see an airplane, make the appropriate sound effects and say that the airplane flies. Do the same with a dog or a fire engine or anything else. If you happen to be outside with your child and see an automobile moving, watch it together and imitate its sound. When you're back home, take out her toy automobile and repeat the process. Use your child's familiar toys and objects and show her how they work. For example, demonstrate that the doll can sit, stand, or lie down, and her truck can move and make sounds.

Blocks. These are ideal for creative play. Your child will be able to arrange blocks in groups (sorting them) according to their size, shape, and color, and will build block towers with considerable skill and imagination. As an example of what you can do, take two red blocks and two green blocks and show her the difference in color. Then take one of the red blocks and ask her to give you the other red block. Although she will not be able to name the actual color, she can learn about different colors at this age. Similarly, you can ask for blocks of the same size or for the little block, and on and on.

Crayons, pencils, and paper. Your baby now is a great scribbler, and with practice can learn to imitate a pretty straight line and sometimes can even make a reasonable attempt at imitating a circle. All this is excellent preparation for her school work later on. Don't expect too much. Remember, penmanship does not count yet.

Mechanical skills. It has been my experience that many parents do not pay enough attention to this area of development. Your child now has the ability and ambition to learn all sorts of mechanical skills. She can be taught to turn on television sets, computers, radios, and light switches. She can learn to put coins into laundromat machines and parking meters and should be taught to buckle her own seat belt. These are all useful skills and improve her manual dexterity as well as give her feelings of participation. Handling a simple record player with an on-and-off-switch mechanism is well within the mechanical capabilities of most eighteen- to twenty-four-month-olds. Pressing elevator buttons is something you can allow your youngster to do that will immediately reward her. The elevator will move because of her skill in button pushing, and she will know it. Of course, unless she is pretty tall for her age, it will be necessary for you to lift her to the level of the elevator buttons. I remember driving across the Triboro Bridge when our son was about two years old and I thought that he was ready to throw the quarter (the tolls were much cheaper in those days) into the basket at the toll booth. He gave it a good try but missed badly. We had sense enough not to criticize him for his wild pitch. He was more successful in throwing the quarter into the basket six months later and he has a perfect record after that. "Easy Pass" has just about eliminated this activity.

Memory. Since your child's memory is improving so dramatically, you should give her every opportunity to develop it. For example, read her a story; then, a couple of hours later, ask her a question about the story, such as, "How did the dog bark?" Children at this age are excellent imitators and mimics of things they have seen or heard. Don't expect your child to remember the details of a story that you may have read to her three days earlier – although I must admit, some of these little children have memories like steel traps and never seem to forget anything. Memory, like everything else, varies from child to child, so I would advise you not to compare your child's memory with that of the child next door.

Hide and seek. Since now your child can actually picture objects and locations in her head, hide-and-seek games can be played on a more sophisticated level. She will be able to look for hidden or missing toys and will not give up easily as before. These hide-and-seek games are best played with other children. Some physiologists believe that understanding the concept that something hidden or missing can be found makes it easier for your child to accept you leaving her on occasion. This is because she will not worry so much that you won't ever come back. I honestly do not know whether or not this is true. I do know that hide-and-seek games give little children a great deal of pleasure, and besides, they are good learning experiences.

Television. I have already made my position clear about television at this age, but now I want to hedge a little. Many parents tell me that their eighteen- to twenty-four-month-olds do seem to enjoy watching short segments of selected children's programs. An occasional viewing of one of these programs may be a good listening and learning experience for some children at this age, and you can try some of the activities performed on these programs with your youngster. However, basically I still believe that most children get very little out of television-watching until they are past two years of age. The large-scale study of more than 3,000 infants and toddlers discussed earlier found that twenty-two percent of one- to two- year-olds watched more than three hours of T.V. each day. This is quite disturbing. So if your toddler is watching and enjoying T.V., make certain that the content of the programs is appropriate (no cartoons) and the maximum T.V. time should not be over one hour per day.

Laughter. Why am I including laughter in this section on mental rather than emotional development? It really belongs in both, but I have chosen to put it here to emphasize the importance of laughter in terms of intellectual achievement. Dr. Abner Ziz, an Israeli psychologist, conducted a three-year study. He concluded that people retain better what they are taught when the teacher uses humor. Laughter helps learning at any age. I always keep this in mind when teaching medical students or pediatric residents. A happy environment full of laughter is the ideal location for optimal learning.

LANGUAGE

We have already discussed the crucial importance of language and what you can expect from your child at this age. To repeat, by two years of age many children have a vocabulary of twenty words, and at times up to fifty words, and understand up to several hundred different words and phrases.

Talking. The key to achieving verbal competence is talking to your child and listening to what she says without interrupting her. If you are not certain what she has said, don't ignore it; rather, ask her to repeat it. A language characteristic of this age is rapid jabbering, called jargon. The avalanche of words that pour out of a child's mouth are full of expressions that have no meaning for you. Some call this jabbering "verbal diarrhea," but I don't particularly like that expression because it has the connotation of a put-down. Jargon is important and you should not be upset or tell your child to slow down her talking. Jargon is a prelude to the next stage, understandable language, and all children have to go through it.

Don't criticize your child's words but rather repeat the word or words correctly, and don't get into the habit of using baby talk. You should ask her for various objects; for example, say, "Show me the red block." Talk to her about such characteristics of objects as top and bottom, heavy or light, wet or dry, hot or cold, and the light. This is the way you can best give your child the words that she will then be able to use to articulate her ideas and thoughts. This is what verbal competence is all about.

Reading. There are many excellent storybooks you can read to your child. Don't be surprised if she prefers to hear the same story over and over again. There is no question that verbal competence is difficult to achieve without a good deal of reading. And don't forget to continue the bedtime reading ritual. Books with large pictures are required at this age. Point to a picture and explain what it is and what it does, or have her point to a picture and then tell her all about it. One of the best ways to ensure that your child will do better in school later on is to help her develop language skills now.

In order to keep this whole discussion of language development in proper perspective, I'd like to quote what the mother of a fine twenty-two-month-old told me recently in my office. "John's working vocabulary is a grand total of three words, but he understands pretty much everything that is spoken to him." About his sparse vocabulary she had this to say: "When he's ready, he's ready." I cannot agree more with what his most intelligent mother said. There is just so much you can do to help your child talk, and no more. When she's ready, the words will come.

Happy second birthday!

Two to Three Years

You can expect an amazing and exciting year. There will be significant advances in your child's physical development, but you will see tremendous advances in both his social and intellectual development.

The two- to three-year-old will begin to construct a new world on the level of verbalization and representation. With his rapidly advancing language skills and his growing ability to think on a symbolic level, he is in a much stronger position to learn about and master more and more of the world around him. Because children of this age can talk and reason and understand, many parents make the serious mistake of pushing them too hard by trying to teach them more than they can handle. The trick is to allow and encourage your child to do as many tasks as he is able without trying to rush him too fast into the adult world. You should always keep in mind that many two- to three-year-olds' mental processes are still quite immature, and they continue to make many errors in their reasoning. For example, a child at this age still believes that anything that moves is alive. Logical reasoning takes many years to master, so it is important that you not expect too much from your child at this age and not overburden him with problems that he is not yet capable of solving.

As I discussed in the previous chapter, a balanced approach is the best one to take. Too much pressure on your baby to learn how to speak or to solve problems will not only slow down his intellectual progress but will also surely lead to difficulties in his emotional development. As Dr. Burton White writes in *The First Three Years of Life,* "...intellectual superiority is very frequently obtained at the expense of progress in other areas of equal or even greater importance."

Quoting from T. Berry Brazelton, a leading child-development expert, "Intelligence is based on emotional adequacy" and I am with him all the way on this. I have already discussed how important it is to help instill self-confidence and self-esteem in your little child but it bears repeating now. Learning numbers, letters, colors, and shapes is much less important than learning to share, interact with others and follow instructions. A child who feels good about himself has the spirit and drive to learn without the fear of failure. Such a child will take some risks in order to learn.

Another cornerstone of intellectual achievement is the child's ability to master symbolic thinking. In *Piaget's Theory of Intellectual Development,* by Herbert Ginsburg and Sylvia Opper, the definition of symbolic thinking is given as the ability to make a mental symbol, an object, or a word represent something else that is not present at that time. These authors give as an example of symbolic thinking a two- to three-year-old who can make a mental symbol or picture of a bicycle or the word "bicycle" or a small schematic toy of a bicycle stand for the real bicycle when it is not in immediate view. This advanced thinking ability allows the child to operate on new and expanded levels. He no longer is restricted to act only upon objects he can see because he now can use a metal picture to remember what he has learned in the past. Because he can now form a mental picture of a bicycle, he is in a position to remember his previous experiences with bicycles.

Symbolic play (make-believe play) is essential for your child's emotional stability and for his ability to adjust to reality. Children between two and three years of age spend a good deal of their time in symbolic play. You should encourage this type of play since your child can use make-believe play to act out the conflicts of his real life in such a way as to make sure he comes out the winner. In real life he often comes out the loser because there are many things he wants that he cannot get and many thoughts he wants to express that he is not yet capable of expressing. More time for playing by himself is needed. His sense of wonder should be encouraged.

There is one word that best describes the basic characteristic of the two- to three-year-old, and that word is "egocentric." By egocentric we mean that the child sees and understands the world entirely and exclusively from his own point of view. I recall a conversation with a mother who could not understand why two-and-a half-year-old Walter was so selfish. "Why can't he understand that I accidentally hit him on the side of his head while I was reaching for one of his toys?" I explained to her that the concept of an "accident" is beyond a two-and-a-half-year-old's comprehension. All little Walter knew was that he was hit on the side of his head by his mother and this understandably made him very angry. I might add that unfortunately many of us remain just as totally self-centered and egocentric throughout life as Walter, not a happy thought.

By the time they reach age two, some children are already "spoiled" and difficult to live with. These youngsters are often angry and hostile and not very lovable much of the time. I will be discussing the subject of anger in some detail in the section on emotional development. Although some of your child's personality traits may already be fairly well-established, you can still do much to mold the positive attributes of his personality and minimize his negative traits. The good news about two- to three-year-olds is that many become less negative than they were at eighteen to twenty-four months of age; if this is the case in your house, be grateful. You can take some of the credit, but don't rest on your laurels.

During this year, children are better able to play alongside other children, and this type of parallel play should be encouraged. This better prepares them for the next step, which is cooperative play. However, do not expect your child at this age to engage in active play with other children (cooperative play). That will not really start until he is over three years old. Since most children of the age enjoy playing by themselves, at times for relatively long periods, some parents assume that they will also play peacefully and contentedly with and alongside another child or two. Not so. If these little children are, in fact, allowed to play together in an unsupervised situation, chaos and destruction are sure to follow. Take my advice when I tell you that play involving your toddler and other children should always be supervised.

By and large these twelve months are a happy and exciting time for your child. Even though he is self-centered and thinks only about himself and is only interested in his own instant gratification and so is often frustrated, he also is very resilient and bounces right back if given half a chance. At this age he is physically able to run, jump, and climb, he can now verbalize many of his needs, and he learns to carry on a two-way conversation. He remains full of energy and enthusiasm. He still takes great pride in his personal accomplishments, and you should continue to praise him for his efforts. This raises an interesting question related to the building up of his self-esteem. Some parents are so caught up with this part of their child's emotional development that they don't take into consideration what the child has actually accomplished. There is a limit to how much you should praise your child. It is counterproductive to make a big fuss over every trivial deed. Both you and your child will know when he really does something worthwhile, and those are the times to tell and show him how proud you are of his success. I am not suggesting that you should not react positively to his accomplishments, but rather that you be somewhat selective when praising him. This approach will motivate him to do his very best and not be content just to coast along on his previous achievements. It will also better prepare him to compete later on in school, where there is no such thing as unrealistic praise.

You will notice that your child is now even more attuned and sensitive to everything that is going on around him. He does not miss a thing. Mr. and Mrs. B., a devoted and loving couple, were the proud parents of three-year-old Christopher. Mrs. B. told me about the time her husband came home from work one day so tired and harassed that he was not in any mood to kiss her "hello," something he did every single night. Christopher picked right up on this and ran to his father, quite upset, and said, "Daddy no kiss Mommy." I believe that it is important for parents to show affection toward each other in front of their children. In my experience, many parents often don't. It is almost as if they are trying to hide overt affectionate advances when their children are around. I also think it is important to show kindness, consideration, and thoughtfulness to each other as well as to the child. It is axiomatic that children learn by example: everything you do rubs off on your child. Happy parents raise happy children.

I want to now discuss with you two words that I have not used up to this point: optimism and courage. I have been struck by the fact that most of the really successful people (both children and adults) I have met through the years have had more than their fair share of these two qualities. I am referring to bank presidents, heads of corporations, leading lawyers and physicians, professors, honor students, class presidents, and others who might be characterized as leaders. The majority are both optimistic and courageous in their approach to life. I have discussed this with many educators, and they agree with me that this has also been their observation. The logical conclusion to be drawn from this is that a high level of achievement is more likely to occur when one has these two basic personality traits. Optimism and courage develop in large measure out of a positive self-image and self-esteem, and pessimism and timidity are the inevitable results of a lack of self-confidence. The courage to take risks and not dwell upon and worry about honest mistakes but rather to learn from them and push on optimistically from there is the hallmark of a truly successful, productive person. You, as parents, will play a large role in determining whether your child grows up with enough self-confidence to achieve the very best that is in him. Your child must be given the freedom and opportunity to experiment and make mistakes without feeling guilty. Although I have not previously used the actual words, I have nevertheless focused on giving you the information and recommendations to help your child develop into a courageous and optimistic human being. The rest of this chapter is devoted to the same purpose.

GROWTH AND DEVELOPMENT

PHYSICAL (MOTOR)

2-3 YEARS

- Walks up and down stairs without difficulty.
- Climbs, runs, and jumps with agility and precision.
- Kicks a ball and throws it with some accuracy.
- Good hand/eye coordination.
- Enjoys playing with and manipulating small objects.
- Learns to ride a tricycle.
- Handles crayon and pencil well.
- Scribbles and can copy lines and circles.
- Can feed himself without much difficulty.
- Can carry heavy objects and push and pull with strength.

Note: These charts are based on average ranges of growth and development; many normal babies perform and achieve either sooner or later than indicated.

GROWTH AND DEVELOPMENT

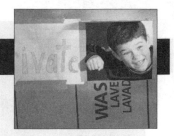

EMOTIONAL (SOCIAL)

2-3 YEARS

- Increased attention span.
- Behavior usually less negative and stubborn.
- Independent; enjoys doing things for himself.
- Great involvement in fantasy or make-believe play.
- Egocentric: sees and understands things completely from his own point of view.
- Enjoys playing alongside other children (not ready for cooperative play).
- Possessive of his belongings but still can be taught to share.
- Spends more time playing away from primary caretaker.
- Sensitive to the feelings of people around him.
- More time spent in role playing.
- Bowel toilet training usually accomplished.
- Enjoys set routine and "rituals" such as bedtime stories.

Note: These charts are based on average ranges of growth and development; many normal babies perform and achieve either sooner or later than indicated.

GROWTH AND DEVELOPMENT

MENTAL (INTELLECTUAL)

2-3 YEARS

- Working vocabulary increases from fifty up to several hundred words by age three.
- Learns to speak short (three- to four-word) sentences that can be understood even by strangers.
- Understands the concept of numbers (one to many).
- Uses "I" instead of his name.
- Can identify many different pictures and objects.
- Answers to and tells you his first (and sometimes his last) name.
- "Hungry" to learn words and meanings.
- Matches some colors.
- Can put on his own shoes but cannot yet tie his laces.
- Follows complicated directions of two or three tasks, one after another.
- Memory greatly improved.
- Symbolic thinking, reasoning, and thoughtfulness more advanced.
- Problem solving improved; enjoys simple puzzles.
- Can build block towers and forts.

Note: These charts are based on average ranges of growth and development; many normal babies perform and achieve either sooner or later than indicated.

PHYSICAL (MOTOR) DEVELOPMENT

Before going on to the physical development of your child I want to discuss four subjects of importance at this age: hearing problems, eye examinations, immunizations, and dental visits.

Hearing problems. It is true that many toddlers are too busy to hear you (selective hearing). Husbands often are guilty of the same problem, especially during football season. However, here are signs of possible hearing loss in your child that you should recognize:

1. A consistent lack of response
2. The inability to follow simple commands
3. Limited understanding and active vocabulary
4. Lack of response to music – no dancing, clapping, or singing along

If you notice any of these signs, call your child's doctor. It may not turn out to be a problem, but it requires medical evaluation. The sooner a hearing loss is discovered, the better the chances of fixing it.

Eye examinations. Even if there is no obvious problem with your child's eyes, such as strabismus (crossed eyes), it is good medical practice for him to have a careful eye examination no later than age two, either by the child's own physician or by an ophthalmologist or optometrist. There is an eye condition called amblyopia (lazy-eye) that can cause a decrease or even loss of vision in the affected eye if not diagnosed early enough. Amblyopia refers to the failure in development of binocular (two-eye) vision, and this results in the child not using one of his eyes to see. If lazy-eye is allowed to progress and continues for too long a period of time without proper treatment, there will be partial or complete loss of vision in the eye that is not being used. The younger the child when the correct diagnosis is made, the better the chance of successful treatment. If caught early enough, treatment is relatively easy and effective. Unfortunately, in many children the problem is not suspected or picked up until they start school and have difficulty reading the blackboard. By then it is usually too late to completely correct the visual defect. It is estimated that four out of one hundred preschool children suffer from ambyopia so it is not an uncommon problem. You may suspect lazy-eye if your child rubs his eyes excessively or shuts or covers one eye to see or tilts his head to one side or blinks frequently. If you notice any of these symptoms it is essential that you notify the child's doctor immediately. Even if he has no noticeable symptoms, he still should have a careful eye examination.

Immunizations. In the birth to three months chapter, I discussed the importance of making sure your child receives all the recommended immunizations on time, a primary series that should be completed by age two. Now is the time to check your records to see if in fact this is the case. As I write this section, two additional vaccines have just been added to the primary series, hepatitis A and rotovirus. If you are not sure about your toddler's immunization status, check with his doctor. If any are missing, arrange for an appointment to complete the series as soon as possible.

Dental visits. Even if your child has no problems with his teeth, he should be taken to a dentist for a routine visit. Some children's dentists recommend that the first visit be at age one. There are two purposes for this check-up:

1. It gets your child accustomed to sitting in the dental chair.

2. It allows the dentist to carefully examine your child's teeth for possible problems and educate you as to the best oral care. The fact is that infections in the mouth can lead to serious infections all over the body.

NUTRITION

By this time your child should be accustomed to feeding himself regular table foods. The diet, it is hoped, has variety, is well-balanced and nutritious, and includes plenty of fruits and vegetables with a minimum of extra salt and sugar. We have already discussed between-meal snacks in the previous chapter. It will now become even more difficult for you to withhold or eliminate junk foods from your child's diet. During this year your child will probably be visiting the homes of other small children, and it is likely that some of their parents are already in the habit of stuffing their youngsters with these non-nutritious, sugar-laden foods. I can assure you that it will not take very long for your child to acquire a strong preference for these sweet junk foods. In addition, you will now be faced with strong competition from your television set regarding food choices, since many two- to three-year-olds become avid T.V. watchers (I will have more to say about television in the sections on exercise and mental development, which follow). A recent task force of the American Psychological Association examined the association between T.V. advertising and the escalating child obesity epidemic. According to their estimate, the average American child watches more than 40,000 T.V. commercials annually. Advertisers spend more than twelve billion dollars per year on ads specifically aimed at children. The products advertised are usually for candy, sugary cereals, soda, and fast foods. Cartoon characters are often used in advertisements for younger children.

Your child will be continuously bombarded with these types of commercials, and as far as a child is concerned, everything he hears on television is true. He will start to tell you what foods he wants you to buy, and most of the time he will ask for foods that he has seen and heard about on television. I had an interesting time talking about the subject of junk food television advertising when I appeared on the "Today" show discussing my first book, *Growing Up Thin*. I remember saying that I had yet to see a television commercial for carrots! That was many years ago and I still am waiting.

Although it won't be easy, it is important that you stand firm and not give in to pressure from your child to buy junk foods. The danger in eating too many junk foods is that they crowd out other nutritious foods. These junk foods kill anyone's appetite for wholesome and nourishing foods. If you have the physical well-being of your child in mind, as I am sure you do, avoid buying these junk foods. They should not be readily available to your child each day.

Between two and three years of age, the improved lines of verbal communication between you and your child may lead to many faulty feeding practices. Many parents use junk food as a reward for good behavior. "If you finish your string beans, you can have a candy bar." "If you stop throwing your toys all over the room, Mommy will give you a piece of cake." Yet another favorite line is, "If you really love Mommy, you will finish all your spinach." There are better ways to reward a child for good behavior than bribing him with unhealthy foods. The attitudes expressed here are all wrong. A child should not eat to please his parents, nor should he eat to get a reward. The only reason he should eat is to satisfy his hunger and supply his body with the proper nutrients for optimum growth and development.

In my practice I place every child who is two years of age or older, thin or fat, on what is called a "prudent" diet. This basically is the same diet that adults with heart disease or high blood pressure are put on in order to slow down the development of atherosclerosis or hardening of the arteries. Although this type of diet in young children has not as yet been proven to slow down the rate of hardening of the arteries, it no doubt does. Such a diet works for adults, so it makes intuitive good sense that it will work the same way in children − and if so, why not use it? The American Academy of Pediatrics recommends such a diet for all children starting at age two whether or not the toddler is overweight. There is no question that the diet is healthy, well-balanced, relatively low in calories, and low in cholesterol and saturated fats. There is absolutely no harm in putting a child on such a diet. Finally, if a child grows up accustomed to eating such a diet, it is much more likely that he will continue to eat the same type of diet as an adult. Such a diet protects against the early onset of coronary heart disease and high blood pressure. There is everything to gain and nothing to lose and that is why it should be started now.

The following are the main features of the "prudent" diet:

Eggs. Egg yolk is extremely high in cholesterol (one of the risk factors in heart disease), so in order to keep down total cholesterol intake, eggs should be restricted to a maximum of three or four per week.

Low-fat or skim milk. The current recommendations of the Committee on Nutrition of the American Academy of Pediatrics is to switch from whole milk to skim or low-fat milk starting at two years of age, and I agree. Both low-fat and skim milk are just as healthy as whole milk but have fewer calories and less fat. Whether or not your child is overweight, a low-fat milk should always be used.

Meats and fish. Red meats (pork and beef) are high in saturated fats, and organ meats (liver, brain, kidney, sweetbreads) are high in cholesterol and they should not be eaten more than two to three times per week. Instead of red meats and organ meats I would suggest that you feed your child more veal, poultry, and fish.

Sugars. Cut down on the intake of refined and processed sugars. This can easily be done by keeping junk foods (cake, candy, soda, and cookies) out of the house except for special occasions like birthday parties.

Salt. It is not necessary to add salt to food since there is plenty of natural salt already there. One accepted method of lowering high blood pressure is to reduce the salt intake. So why get your child used to salty tasting foods? A good idea is to keep saltshakers off the table.

Cereals. Stay away from the extra sugary kinds. If you put some fruit on the various unsugared cereals, they taste fine and are far healthier.

I can almost hear you thinking, "But how can I deprive my little child of all these delicious treats?" An occasional treat is okay, but not as part of the everyday diet. Yes, you may be "depriving" you child by following my suggestions, but what you actually will be "depriving" him of is dental decay, obesity, type 2 diabetes, early onset of heart disease, and high blood pressure. These are all important "deprivations."

If you look at your child and find he is too fat, do not automatically assume that the obesity will go away. The longer you allow him remain fat, the more likely he will be fat all his life. If this is the case in your house, check with his doctor and ask his advice. You will probably have to modify your child's diet and cut down on some calories, as well as increase his physical activity. This is easier do now than later on, when he is more set in his eating and exercise patterns.

The epidemic of childhood obesity has reached crisis proportions. *Growing Up Thin,* published in 1975, was the first book to address the problem of overweight children and what should be done about it. We coined the phrase "fat proof" your house. Sad to say, despite my best efforts in promoting my book and its ideas, the current generation of children is fatter than ever.

It has become abundantly clear that the treatment of childhood, adolescent, and adult obesity rarely is successful. I am convinced that the answer is not treatment but rather prevention. Your job as parents is to prevent your young child from ever becoming fat in the first place. Prevention should start now, especially if one or both parents are overweight. There is a significant genetic component to obesity. If both parents are overweight, there is an eighty percent chance that their child will become obese, and if one parent is overweight, there is a fifty percent chance the child will become obese. These genetic "high risk" families should carefully monitor their child's weight and weight gain, and the earlier this is begun, the better. As the prevalence of childhood obesity has increased (data from The International Obesity Task Force indicated that more than twenty-two million children under five years of age in the United States are overweight or obese) so have the adverse health consequences. These include cardiovascular disease, high blood fat levels, high blood pressure, and type 2 diabetes. These high risk factors, when in combination, are called the Metabolic Syndrome. Thirty percent of overweight teenagers suffer with this dangerous condition, which persists into adulthood. Obesity plays a central role in the development of the Metabolic Syndrome, which makes the prevention and treatment of childhood obesity so very important.

I have had a large experience dealing with the problem of obesity in children through the years. I can assure you that even if both parents are obese, they can raise a normal weight child provided they start early, before he becomes fat. The proper diet and exercise program, under your child's doctor's supervision can be successful. The key to success is to start early, which means right now.

I would suggest that you do not waste your time trying to teach your child good table manners at this age. It just won't work. What you can do is set a proper example in terms of how you eat, and that is all. If you eat slowly, always sit down while you eat, and chew your food slowly, chances are that your child will eventually learn to eat the same way. The entire family should eat together whenever possible, and every member should be served the same "prudent" type of diet described above.

Continue to prevent your child from becoming iron-deficient. His brain is still growing rapidly and needs the iron to develop normally. As I pointed out earlier, iron-deficiency, especially during the first three years of life, is associated with impaired mental development and increased absorption of lead from the environment, also resulting in lost I.Q. points, as stated earlier. In our office, we advise a daily iron-fortified multi-vitamin for every toddler. If your child has not been taking an iron-fortified vitamin, discuss this with his doctor.

More and more evidence continues to accumulate demonstrating how important proper nutrition is in terms of overall health and longevity. I believe that it is never too early to start your child on the road to correct eating. The facts are that too many of us, both children and adults, consume unhealthy diets, too high in saturated fat, sugar, salt, junk food, and calories.

EXERCISE

Little children at this age love to run, jump, climb, and balance themselves. They can be taught to ride a tricycle and greatly enjoy all sorts of rhythmic play and dancing. They try very hard to exercise their large muscles by involving themselves in all sorts of vigorous activities. If you give your child the opportunity, he will happily spend many hours each day in an excellent continuing program of physical fitness. However, our culture makes it difficult for youngsters to exercise to the degree required to develop and maintain optimal physical fitness. The many work-saving conveniences that eliminate physical effort – the automobile, elevator, and escalator   all lead to a sedentary lifestyle. If you add to these factors the lack of encouragement to exercise in early life, the result is that many of our preschool children are not given sufficient opportunity to challenge their musculoskeletal systems and so cannot achieve real physical vigor and well-being. Television plays an important part in interfering with proper physical development. A child at this age who becomes accustomed to sitting in front of the television set for hours on end (often with a sugar-laden snack to keep him company) will undoubtedly continue to behave this way as he grows older. The results are obvious. By the time these inactive children are ready for school, they are already flabby, overweight, poorly coordinated, and unable to keep up with their more physically fit classmates. A recent large-scale study clearly showed that watching T.V. for over two hours a day greatly increased the risk of obesity.

If you don't want this to happen to your child, the time to do something about it is now. Encourage your child to exercise every chance he gets. Let him walk rather then ride in a car and walk up the stairs with you rather than take the elevator or escalator. Keep his television watching to no more than one hour a day, and of course, be selective in what he watches (more about this in the mental development section). The Committee on Public

Education of the American Academy of Pediatrics recommends that T.V. watching for children over two years of age be limited to no more than one to two hours of quality programming per day. According to an interesting statistic that I came across, the average American child spends more time watching television (15,000 hours) than in the classroom (11,000 hours). A recent American Academy of Pediatrics statement cites Neilsen ratings showing that two- to-three-year-olds watch an average of twenty-five hours of T.V. each week.

Parents who truly have their children's best interests at heart must set proper examples. The sedentary, inactive lifestyle of the majority of adults in our society teaches their children that it is also perfectly acceptable for them to sit around much of the time. A survey conducted by the President's Council on Physical Fitness reflects this sorry state of affairs. This study showed that forty-five percent of all adult Americans do not engage in any physical activity for the purpose of exercise. Even more significant is the fact that most of these nonexercisers believe that they are getting enough exercise. If you fall into this group of nonexercisers, my advice is to change your ways, not only for your own health and well-being but also for your child's.

The Committee on Pediatric Aspects of Physical Fitness, Recreation and Sports of the American Academy of Pediatrics has pointed out a major flaw in our present system of health care. The emphasis in evaluating the health of a child is primarily on the presence or absence of disease, with little regard given to the quality of how he functions. An infant or child is considered healthy if he is fully immunized and free of any specific illness. This definition of optimal health is not complete. As part of the overall evaluation of the health status of the child, we should also ask and determine if he is able to meet his daily tasks, activities, and sudden emergencies with enthusiasm and vigor and without tiring too quickly. I believe that a child so out of shape that he can't keep up with his peers is just as unhealthy as if he was suffering from a particular illness.

Before going on to recommend specific exercises and activities for your two- to three-year-old, I want to call your attention to another important reason for encouraging your child to exercise (and to exercise more yourself). Many investigations have clearly demonstrated that exercise lowers both cholesterol levels and blood pressure. Further, exercise strengthens the heart muscles by increasing the collateral circulation to the heart. All this means that exercise protects against heart attacks. I once gave this lecture to an obese mother and father of a fat two-and-a-half-year-old. When I finished, Mr. A. responded with, "I can understand what you are saying about my wife and myself but, Dr. Eden, you certainly don't mean that Eric will get a heart attack if he doesn't exercise." Obviously, two- to three-year-olds don't suffer heart attacks, but if Eric does not start exercising soon, it is unlikely that he will ever become physically fit or normal weight, so he will in fact be at greater risk of developing a heart attack or stroke as an adult. I am happy to report that his family took my advice seriously and are all in better shape than ever. More and more toddlers are spending their time doing nothing but sitting in front of T.V. sets. Dr. William Wilkoff, writing in *Pediatric News* in January 2007, finds that fewer children in his practice nowadays are active enough to sustain bumps and bruises as compared to years ago. He writes "couch potatoes only get bruised if they fall off their chairs onto the floor."

SPECIFIC RECOMMENDATIONS

The following are the physical activities, exercises, and equipment that will help your child achieve real physical fitness.

Climbing equipment. We have already discussed this in previous chapters. I just want to add here that the two- to three-year-old is fascinated by this type of equipment, as well as by swings and slides. Playing on all these is splendid exercise. It strengthens his muscles and helps build up his coordination and agility. I would strongly recommend that these activities always be supervised to prevent serious accidents.

Toy wheelbarrows and construction trucks. Carrying and dumping sand, dirt, and toys is what a two- to three-year-old enjoys more than anything else. This is another fine way for him to develop his large muscles. It also is a form of make-believe play in that he imagines he really is working.

Tricycle. Now is the time for you to supply your child with a tricycle. Between two and three years of age most children can be taught to use the pedals. After he masters this new skill, you will find it difficult to keep your child off his tricycle. This is good exercise for developing good leg muscles and coordination. Again, make certain that he rides his tricycle on the sidewalks and in safe places. If not specifically warned over and over again, a child will take off into traffic. Your toddler should always wear a helmet while riding. This is essential for his safety. Helmets prevent most head injuries, according to data from the United States Consumer Product Safety Commission and the National Pediatric Trauma Registry. The use of helmets early on will also help form habits that result in improved helmet use as young cyclists grow older.

Toy tools and a toy workbench. We have already discussed this. It is an excellent way to let off steam, burn up calories, and exercise. It is also useful for developing good hand-eye coordination.

Coloring books. I have included coloring books because coloring is an activity that improves hand-eye coordination.

Pulling wagons, large balls, and large blocks. All these help your child's large-muscle development.

Sports. This is a good age to encourage the development of skills in various sports activities, especially those that your child can continue all his life. It is a bit too early to think about skiing, skating, bowling, tennis, or golf, but how about swimming, running, and soccer? Two- to three-year-olds can be taught to swim since they have no fear of the water. It is important that they not be rushed and that the instruction be supervised by an expert. Many YMCAs and other organizations have programs designed specifically to teach little children to swim. Some parents worry about chlorine in the pools. In my experience, this is seldom a problem.

Soccer is becoming very popular in the United States, and since a two- to three-year-old can kick a ball and run all day, it is an ideal sport for him. Your child probably can throw a ball and learn to catch one now. Throwing and catching with your child helps promote physical fitness and coordination. It improves hand-eye coordination and, of course, his actual skill in learning to throw and catch. When he reaches Little League age, he will have a better chance of excelling. Don't neglect wrestling, great fun and an excellent overall conditioner. It builds up strength, agility, and balance.

SAFETY TIPS

A two- to three-year-old child is extremely active and his actions are often unpredictable. Although he understands quite a bit, he still does not have the judgment or the experience to realize what is dangerous. In order to prevent accidents and injuries, your child needs your supervision and protection and some rules of behavior he can follow.

In the automobile. More than fifteen hundred children under four years of age die each year from automobile accidents. Most of these deaths are preventable. The great majority of preschool-age children ride in cars without using any type of safety restraint. Studies have proven that both death and injury rates can be reduced by over eighty percent if a child seat restraint is used. You must make sure that your child wears an approved automobile child restraint every time he rides in a car. Always put him in the back seat. This is the safest place in the car since its further away from a head-on crash, the most common type of collision.

Dogs. Here are some points to remember about dogs:
1. Never leave your toddler alone with any dog, whether it be a strange one or your own loyal, friendly, lovable animal.
2. Teach your child not to play with a dog while he is eating and not to suddenly wake a sleeping dog.
3. Teach him to stay away from strange dogs.
4. Always contact your child's doctor if your child gets bitten by a dog or any animal when the skin is broken, however minor the injury appears.

Play injuries. Always check all your child's toys and playground equipment for sharp edges and small, easily swallowed parts. Tricycles and riding toys should only be used on sidewalks.

Fires and burns. This is the third-ranking cause of accidental death in children between one and thirteen years of age. Therefore make it a habit always to keep matches and cigarette lighters away from children. Purchase flame-retardant sleepwear for your child and don't allow your young child to turn on hot-water faucets.

Drowning. I have said this earlier but let me repeat it: Never leave your child alone in a bathtub, or in any other water, for that matter. If your child is on a boat with you, he should always wear his own flotation device. A statistic to keep in mind is that an average of twenty-five hundred children die each year in the United States as a result of drowning.

Falls and cuts. Store your scissors and knives out of sight and out of reach of your child. When possible, use safety-glass doors. Install guards on all windows, especially those above the first floor as well as stairway gates.

Dangerous objects. Always lock up dangerous tools and garden equipment. Keep your little child away from lawn mowers and power tools. I have seen many serious accidents involving both lawn mowers and power tools.

Lyme disease. Your active toddler will be spending more time outdoors and so may be exposed to tick bites. Here are some tips to prevent lyme disease when he is outside playing in wooded areas:
1. He should wear long-sleeved shirts tucked into his pants and long pants tucked into his socks.
2. Spray his clothing with an insect repellent containing DEET.

3. Most important of all is to carefully check him from head to toe for ticks each night before going to bed. It takes twenty-four to forty-eight hours of tick attachment to transmit the disease, so finding and removing a tick less than twenty-four hours after attachment prevents lyme disease. If you do this, you have nothing to worry about.

4. Never hold and squeeze the tick. Rather, use a fine tweezer to grab the tick by the head area where it entered the skin and pull up firmly without twisting. Clean the bite area with a disinfectant.

Poisons. I covered this subject in detail in the previous chapter. You must continue to be on the alert since the incidence of poisoning remains high in the two- to three-year-old group. A few more words about lead poisoning: Toddlers are particularly at high risk from increased lead absorption because of their increased hand to mouth activity, increased lead absorption from the gastrointestinal tract, and the vulnerability of their developing central nervous system. Indeed, studies have shown that the highest blood levels in all age groups are found in two year olds. Lead paint was banned in the United States in 1978, so if you live in a pre-1978 house beware of deteriorating or peeling paint and plaster. The most common pathway of lead exposure today is through ingestion of house dust contaminated with lead coming from deteriorated paint and tracked-in soil. The soil contains lead from past leaded gasoline and weathering of lead containing paint. If your child enjoys eating dirt, check his blood lead level. Continue his iron-fortified vitamin to prevent iron-deficiency. Remember that iron increases the amount of lead absorbed.

Most injuries are preventable. They usually result from inadequate supervision, carelessness, or an improperly child-proofed home. If you keep these safety tips in mind, your child will be much less likely ever to suffer a serious or catastrophic accident or injury.

EMOTIONAL (SOCIAL) DEVELOPMENT

There are five important general areas related to the emotional development of the two- to three-year-old that I want to discuss before going on to list specific recommendations. These topics, all crucial in terms of your child's future personality, are toilet training, anger, fears, body image, and the birth of another child.

TOILET TRAINING

I believe that most children are ready to be trained at around two years of age, give or take a few months. It has been my experience that a great many parents are overly concerned and worried about what is in reality a simple and normal developmental process. It must be remembered that properly achieved toilet training is a great source of satisfaction for your child. Some children train themselves. Others require and deserve your help and guidance. The most important factor in toilet training is your attitude. Sixty to seventy years ago many children were completely toilet trained by one year of age, and in many cases this was the result of rigid and at times coercive methods. We have since learned that these techniques sometimes resulted in psychological problems for the child later on. Therefore, in recent years the pendulum has swung in the opposite direction. Many parents now take what I consider an overly permissive attitude to toilet training and say, "Leave him alone; he will train himself when he is ready." Those in this laissez-faire group are afraid that any active intervention on their part will cause their child to become angry and hostile.

My position regarding toilet training is middle-of-the-road. I believe that the answer lies somewhere between total permissiveness and the unyielding, rigid approach of yesteryear. The proper approach to toilet training (and, incidentally, toward almost everything else related to your child) should be one of friendliness, encouragement, and interest, along with consistency and perseverance. Taking such a posture will not frustrate your child, nor will it allow the situation to get completely out of hand. On the contrary, this supportive attitude will help encourage your child to please you and will ultimately play an important part in building up self-esteem and the vital, trusting bond between you that is so very important. Try to make toilet training fun rather than a battle.

By age two, most children have some regularity in their bowel movements and also are aware of when they are about to move their bowels. This is the right time to start the toilet-training process. All you need to do is learn to recognize the warning signs your baby gives before defecating; the rest is simple. Now is the time to get out his potty chair and sit him down when he gives you the proper signal. You can also use a baby seat on the regular toilet seat (this takes up less room than a potty chair) as long as there is a foot rest so that his feet don't dangle. An encouraging, optimistic approach works best. It may take weeks and sometimes months before he is successful for the first time. When that red-letter day finally arrives, make a big fuss about it. Tell him how proud and happy you are of his accomplishment and what a big boy he is. It takes a great deal of patience on your part, but try to remember that you are not working against any deadline. Never chastise or yell at or punish him, and above all else never shame him when he fails. There is no reason to compete with your neighbor in terms of who gets their child trained first. Some children take longer than others to train – and so what? It is counterproductive in terms of your child achieving emotional stability and self-confidence if you make him feel guilty when he does not succeed. I have taken care of many children, including my own two, who were not yet trained as they sat down proudly to cut their third birthday cakes, still wearing diapers under their party clothes. Take my word for it – they both became toilet trained soon after, and both became physicians much later on.

MYTH: Late toilet training is associated with low intelligence.

This is not true. As I wrote in *Handbook for New Parents*, "...there is absolutely no relationship between late toilet training and lack of intelligence. [Your child] can still grow up to be a professor at M.I.T."

I have not discussed bladder training, since successful bowel training usually results in the simultaneous control of urination. Therefore, most of the time it is not necessary to do much about urine training. Two suggestions that you may find helpful in achieving urine control are, first, wait for your child to be dry for about two hours and then take him to the potty chair. Also, use training pants. A two-year-old child usually does not like a cold, wet diaper, and transferring to training pants at the age of two can act as a stimulus for more speedy training. Boys are usually slower than girls in establishing control of their urine. Just as with bowel-movement training, there will be many accidents with urination. Sooner or later your child will be successful. Nighttime bladder control comes last, and you should do nothing about it. Once again, time and patience will take care of this.

The process of toilet training should be thought of as a natural event in your child's life and of considerable importance to his normal emotional development. Properly helping him to succeed when he is able will help you establish a strong, positive bond with your child. It will do a world of good in building up his self-esteem and self-image. An interested, friendly, consistent, and encouraging attitude is the key. You do not have to read entire books devoted to how to toilet train your child. As a matter of fact, I was recently asked by a publisher if I would be interested in writing the complete guide to toilet training. I thanked him for thinking of me, but turned him down. All you need is common sense and a good approach.

ANGER

Handling your child's anger and aggression and disobedience at this age can be both difficult and distressing. Many of us were never taught how to handle anger during our own childhood. We have been made to believe that anger is bad and so we automatically feel guilty when we are angry, even if the anger is justified. If we could get rid of this notion once and for all, it would make it easier for us to deal with our children's angry outbursts and aggressive behavior. The goal really should not be to repress these angry feelings in our children but rather to accept these feelings as a fact of life and help channel them toward constructive and positive goals instead.

In order for you to be able to respond sensibly to anger and aggression in your child, you must first understand some of the feelings within the child that trigger this behavior. His anger may be associated with failure or frustration, a feeling of lowered self-esteem, loneliness, and neglect, or it may be related to anxiety. Anger may be associated with sadness, jealousy, depression, or feelings of overdependency and frustration. It is important to remember that little children have the very same feelings that we do. The difference is that the little child is not yet mature enough to handle many of these feelings except by expressing anger, aggression, and negative behavior. I might add that there are lots of adults who have never matured beyond this childish response.

As I already suggested in a discussion on discipline in a previous chapter, it is much better to try to teach your child right from wrong than to automatically punish him for his negative behavior. Always punishing a child when he is aggressive or angry is the wrong way to communicate to him what you really expect. Your child must be taught more acceptable methods of coping with and handling his anger. As I mentioned earlier, discipline means teaching rather than punishing.

Good discipline involves creating an atmosphere of firmness, fairness, and reason. Bad discipline represents harsh and inappropriate punishment. Approach and accept your angry or disobedient child as a human being with a problem. He has feelings that he must express one way or another.

Before giving you some good discipline techniques for dealing with your angry disobedient child, I would like discuss a widely used inappropriate technique – spanking or hitting your toddler.

First some statistics taken from an article by Dr. Barbara Howard, a behavioral pediatrician at John's Hopkins University Department of Pediatrics. Over seventy percent of parents, both mothers and fathers, hit their one year olds, and ninety percent of three-year-olds get spanked. Toddlers misbehave every six to eight minutes so it is not surprising that there will be a lot of hitting if corporal punishment is a big part of the parents' disciplinary repertoire. Further, as the child get older, it will get worse.

Hitting your child may work for the moment, but the facts are that kids who are spanked become more aggressive, less attentive, more likely to have delinquent behavior outside the home, and more likely to become a spouse abuser than children who are not hit. How much does spanking increase the risk of a child becoming aggressive? It doesn't always happen, but research shows that there may be a fourfold increase.

Finally, I want you to understand that painful punishments will make other nonpainful punishment less effective. A "time out" in preschool for a child who has been hit at home is a piece of cake. By spanking your child at home you will be making it more difficult for the school to manage your child.

Hitting your child is psychologically damaging and not productive. Other poor discipline techniques include excessive screaming and yelling, empty promises, and ridiculous threats.

There will be times when you probably will be unable to control yourself and will lash out at your misbehaving toddler inappropriately. Nobody is perfect, but if you keep these episodes to a minimum, all will be well.

The following are suggestions, some of which I have already written about, for dealing with the angry and disobedient child.

Promises and rewards. These are much more effective than punishment. Always remember to keep your promises, and as a rule, don't use food as one of the rewards.

Scene removal. This method of discipline should not be viewed strictly as punishment, but rather as your way of saying to your child that his behavior at the time is unacceptable and therefore he must leave the scene. I would suggest that you save this method for important occasions such as, for example, when he is about to hurt himself or somebody else or when he is having a temper tantrum at the supermarket. It is a good idea to make sure that your child is fed and rested before you go out. Hunger and fatigue can make a child more tantrum prone. To be at all effective, you should calmly separate him from the scene of the crime, without losing your own temper. If you are consistent, he will soon get the message.

Time out. This can be an effective discipline technique used at home when things are getting out of hand. It involves time away from the scene of the episode, along with signs of disapproval on your part and temporary loss of freedom and loss of interesting things for your child to do. A brief time on a designated chair or on the bed in his room, during which you pay no attention to him, can work very well. How long should the time out be? One minute is too short, and twenty years is too long. Five minutes seems about right. For your toddler the five minutes seems like an eternity.

Explanations. The two- to-three-year-old child understands much of what you say to him. Help him understand the cause of his angry or aggressive behavior. It is amazing how quickly a child will react properly if he understands what actually frustrated him, especially if you do your explaining quickly and sympathetically.

Let the punishment fit the crime. Let your child know the consequences of his behavior ahead of time. If he needs discipline, try to make it relate to the situation in order to teach him a lesson. For example, sending him to bed for throwing his toys all over the house makes no sense. Rather, forbidding him from playing with his toys for awhile will help him better understand the problem.

Listening. Encourage your child to talk about his bad feeling. For example, if he hurts his hand, ask him to tell you about it. The verbal group of two-to three-year-olds find this approach useful. This method probably is more effective after the child is three years old and a better talker.

Be sympathetic. Get into the habit of telling your child when he is acting up that you understand his feelings of anger and frustration. Tell him that instead of screaming and hitting, you would like him to tell you in words what is bothering him. As he gets closer to age three, he will be better able to respond appropriately to this approach.

Don't be afraid to say "no." It is important that you set limits, clearly explain them to your child, and then stick to your word. He must understand that you will not tolerate unacceptable or antisocial behavior. If your two- to three-year-old insists on riding his tricycle out into the street despite your repeated warning, it is time to stop reasoning with him. Giving him a firm smack across his backside (this is my only exception to the anti-hitting rule) and then taking the tricycle away for a few days will be much more effective. I do not consider this child abuse. On the contrary, it is simply a preventive technique for survival.

Fears. All children develop fears of one kind or another. You cannot prevent them, but you can help overcome them. Here are three of the most frequent fears seen at this age and what you can do about them:

1. Separation: It is normal for your child to worry when you leave. Always tell him when you will be back. Introduce him slowly to any new caretaker and explain that this person will take care of him until you get back home.

2. Doctors: This is a real fear because the doctor so often inflicts pain with all the shots he gives in order to fully immunize him. A good idea is to use a play doctor kit to show him what will happen. It also helps if you have a friendly pediatrician who spends a little time talking to him before stabbing him with a sharp needle.

3. The dark: In a way, this is a form of separation anxiety. The way to handle it is to establish a regular bedtime routine (which should have been established earlier) and put in a nightlight. A stuffed animal may also help.

Other common fears are the fear of sudden loud noises, death, animals, and toilet training.

Try to accept any and all of his fears as being very real to him. These fears are not signs of impaired emotional development. They should never be ignored or laughed off. When appropriate, take him away from the frightening situation and after calming him down, talk to him about it and listen as he tries to express his feelings to you.

BODY IMAGE

Another aspect of building up self-esteem involves helping your child develop a positive body image by learning to admire and love his own body. Without a healthy body image it will be much more difficult for him to establish real feelings of self-worth and self-esteem. I believe that one of the important goals of all parents should be to make every possible effort to help their children feel comfortable and happy about their bodies. Now is not too early to begin. If you are successful in this undertaking, your child will become less vulnerable to other people's estimates of him and therefore less susceptible to possible future embarrassment and shame.

Many children grow up with negative feeling about their bodies, and too often parents are unaware of the adverse psychological consequences that will follow. These children grow up with disturbed and sometimes even distorted images of themselves and inevitably suffer from a lowering of their self-esteem and self-confidence.

There are a number of reasons why so many children end up with negative feelings about their bodies and there are specific steps you can take to prevent this from happening. The first reason is related to our puritanical heritage, with its emphasis on the body as being inherently "dirty" and a source of evil and temptation. The mother who slaps her child's hand when he plays with his penis inadvertently helps to promote negative feelings in the child's mind about that particular "bad" part of his anatomy. Although you may find it difficult to do so (especially in front of company), let your child explore his body without interfering. Teach your child the words for all parts of his body, including his penis and testicles. If you have a girl, teach her the word vagina and not some nonsensical baby word for it. It is amazing how many different ridiculous synonyms are given for vagina and penis. I have been struck by how few parents teach their two- to three-year-olds to use the proper words, but they have no trouble at all with eyes, ears, nose, and mouth. These mothers and fathers cannot accept the fact that those future sexual areas of the body are o.k. to look at and talk about. If, as you read this, you realize that you belong to this "uptight" group, I suggest that you try not to instill these same attitudes in your child. Passing on to your child your perception of him as having a beautiful body, including all his parts, will give him the permission and encouragement to appreciate and become more comfortable with himself. I understand that this is a tall order for some parents, but it is something to seriously think about.

MYTH: Masturbation in a little child is unhealthy, a sign of emotional trouble, or a sign of being oversexed.

Masturbation during the first few years of life is a harmless habit and does not hurt the child in any way. It is normal behavior and does not warrant scolding, punishment, or instilling guilt.

The other main reasons leading to the formation of a negative body image have already been covered in the physical development section of this chapter. One is our sedentary lifestyle, with its lack of exercise. This leads to flabbiness, clumsiness, obesity, and poor muscle tone. Another is related to the foods we eat, a diet too high in calories, fats, and refined sugars. Although a two- to three-year-old who is too fat will not worry about it, if he stays fat long enough, he will eventually face ridicule, shame, and embarrassment as a schoolboy or adolescent. It makes little difference which comes first, the obesity or the negative body image; one goes right along with the other.

Not enough emphasis has been placed on the importance of helping children develop a good feeling about their bodies. There is little question that distorted and disturbed body images lead to emotional difficulties. It is important that you take the necessary steps now to promote a positive body image in your little child. If you succeed, you will have taken a big step in ensuring that he will grow up feeling better about himself and with an increased zest for life.

THE BIRTH OF ANOTHER CHILD

You may have noticed that up until now we have approached the subject of raising your child as if he were an only child. If you have been reading this book as a parent of more than one child, you have already realized how much more difficult it is to give time and attention to your baby with an older sibling or two or three around. If this is the case, you also have had experience dealing with jealousies and conflicts between them. But if you have a two- to three-year-old and are thinking about having another child, or if you are pregnant or have just given birth to a new baby, what I have to say now may be more meaningful.

"Dr. Eden, my Johnny is two-and-a-half years old. Do you think it's a good idea for me to have another baby because we want Johnny to have company?" My answer to that mother was that although it is true that a new baby certainly will be good company for Johnny, that is not in itself a good enough reason for deciding to have another baby. If that is your only reason for wanting another child, I would advise you to reconsider your decision.

"What is the ideal spacing between children?" As far as I am concerned, there is no such thing. While it is true that the rivalry between children who are less than three years apart is often more intense that that between children spaced farther apart, I don't believe that this fact should enter very seriously into your decision. Whatever the age differences between your children, there will always be some jealousy and rivalry. My brother is five-and-a-half years older than me and as I recall, we fought with each other throughout my childhood. My own two children are two-and-a-half years apart and they fought with each other all through their childhoods. Sibling rivalry should be accepted as normal, healthy behavior. It simply represents competition between children. Fighting between siblings can never be eliminated, but it can be minimized if you understand what is going on.

When your two- to three-year-old, without having asked for one, is presented with a baby brother or sister, how will he feel and act, and how should you deal with these feelings and actions?

First of all, he will feel abandoned when his mother leaves him to go to the hospital to have the new baby. It will help if this doesn't come as a complete surprise to him. It is wiser to give him some prior warning about what is going to happen. This reminds me of the mother of a two-and-a-half-year-old boy who visited her obstetrician and was told that she was six weeks pregnant. She could not wait to get home and spring the good news on her son. This is ridiculous; your child does not need that much notice. It is a better idea to wait until one to two months before your delivery date and then tell him about it. Of course, it he notices your changing body shape and asks you why you are becoming so fat, it's time to explain about the new baby. When you do go to the hospital, talk to him about it, and it possible, arrange for him to visit you there. Unfortunately, many hospital maternity units do not allow two- to three-year-old visitors. If this is the case, a good compromise would be to phone him each day from your hospital bed. This will lessen his anxiety and feelings of desertion.

Your child's second normal reaction will be jealousy of all the attention heaped on the new and, from his point of view, unwanted member of the family. I suggest you come home from the hospital with two presents: one, the new baby, and the other, a special toy for your older child. I'll never forget one mother who really took this suggestion seriously. Coming home from the hospital with big brother Joseph waiting expectantly at the front door, mama got out of her car, handed the new baby to her husband and a Labrador retriever to her son. It is also a good idea to keep a number of other presents on hand to give him each time a visitor brings a gift for the new baby.

Third, your child will rightly be upset because you are now spending so much of your time with the new baby. This cannot be helped, and there is no reason to feel guilty about it. Try your best to allocate a separate time away from the new baby for your two- to three-year-old. Since you have already had previous experience with a new baby, you should be more efficient now and better able to find the time. Whenever possible, take him out of the house without the new baby for an automobile ride to the supermarket, to the park, etc. Use these times to remind him that he is the big brother.

Another reaction of your two- to three-year-old will probably be anger and hostility. Accept this as a normal reaction to a situation he does not like. Limits must be set. No matter how angry or jealous he may be, hitting the new baby is completely unacceptable. Tell your child that it is okay to become angry, but hitting and hurting are out. An attuned and sympathetic mother once taught me a constructive way to help handle the jealousy. She made it her business to criticize her new baby from time to time while the older child was around. She would chastise and scold the new baby for such things as having a dirty diaper, crying, refusing his food, and the like, and her older child would carefully observe all this and seem very happy about it. I will never forget what that mother said to me: "If Susan knew the words, she would say, 'Thank God there really is some justice in the world.'"

When another baby is born, your child may regress in his behavior. During my telephone advice hour one morning I heard the following from a flabbergasted mother: "Our new baby has been home exactly three days and Dennis [age two year, nine months] is already back into diapers and stealing the new baby's bottle." I advised this mother and I am advising you not to be concerned about this regressive behavior. If you stop yourself from criticizing your child with such statements as "I am ashamed of you" or "Don't act like a baby," and simply leave him alone, he will quickly revert back to his normal, more mature ways.

Finally, I would advise you to try to involve your two- to three-year-old in helping out with the new baby. He really can be very useful. Tell him how much you and the new baby appreciate his assistance. Showing him how much you appreciate his help and how important he is to you will help reduce his feelings of hostility and jealousy toward the new star attraction.

AUTISM

A few words about the subject of autism are in order. The earlier autism is recognized the better the chance of effective intervention and improved outcome. By two years of age there usually are a number of signs that should alert you to the real possibility that your child may be autistic. These "Red Flag" signs include:

- Not making eye contact
- Not taking any interest in other children
- Preferring to play by himself
- Repetitive motor mannerisms, such as rocking or hand flapping
- Delayed language development (should be using two-word phrases by age two)
- Intense temper tantrums
- Unable to cope with any change in routine

Even if your child demonstrates some of these behavior patterns, it does not mean that he is autistic. The diagnosis is difficult and requires careful professional evaluation since there is no specific diagnostic test for autism. Many perfectly normal children have characteristics that are compatible with some signs of autism.

If you suspect that there may be a problem, discuss it with your child's doctor as soon as possible. Most of the time your suspicions will turn out to be wrong. But, as with pretty much everything, better safe than sorry.

SPECIFIC SUGGESTIONS

The following are my recommendations for some specific activities to help your two- to three-year-old better achieve emotional stability and maturity:

"Dress-up" clothes. This is an excellent activity for make-believe play, and children love it. Take your choice, but mine is hats, all sorts of hats. The more, the merrier! One of the funniest home movies I have ever taken was of our daughter, age two-and-a-half, in our backyard trying on one different hat after another as fast as she could, hamming it up and laughing with glee at each and every change.

Toy trains. Your two- to three-year-old should be ready for toy trains that he can hook together and take apart himself. After you show him how they work, all he needs is a conductor's hat and he is ready to take off (in his mind) on all sorts of wonderful trips. Yes, Dad, it's too early for you to buy him electric trains!

Wooden and plastic blocks. These remain ideal for imaginative and creative play. Your child can build forts and towers and buildings; then he can knock them down and begin all over again.

Finger puppets. Many children in this age group have a great deal of fun with puppets. They can be taught to manipulate them, and it is a fine way for children to exercise their imaginations and creativity.

Painting. Your child can be given a paintbrush or use his fingers or he can use both. I have to admit that finger painting, although a fine outlet for your child to express his feelings, can get pretty messy. If he does finger paint, be sure to spread plenty of newspaper on the floor – and I would advise you not to dress him up in his Sunday finest. In *Teach Your Baby to Talk,* Dr. Pushaw suggests using chocolate pudding on wax paper for finger painting. It sounds like a fine idea. If the child isn't happy with what he has painted, he can eat the chocolate and start all over.

Pasting. This is another messy but useful activity for your child's emotional development. Pasting is similar to painting in that it is an expressive experience for him. It is another way for him to let out his feelings. One easy method to make paste is mixing flour, salt, and water.

Singing. At this age children love to imitate, and they are ready and more than willing to sing along with you. Some favorite songs that you can sing together are "Row, Row, Row Your Boat," "Twinkle, Twinkle, Little Star," and "Jingle Bells."

Dancing. I consider this an important and often neglected activity. Dancing will do wonders for a child's body image, self-expression, and feelings. Also, it is a fine form of exercise. You can make up dances together, dancing in time to the music. Your child can dance to show how he feels. Parents who are not comfortable dancing themselves find this a difficult activity. If you and your child are alone, there is no reason to feel embarrassed. Just relax and let yourself go in time to the music and your child will do the same. Dancing allows a child to become more comfortable with his own body and this good feeling (positive body image) will stay with him as he grows and matures.

Rhythmic instruments. I am referring to pots, pans, and spoons; with these instruments a child has the opportunity to bang away and march around the room to his heart's content. It might be wise to get yourself a set of earplugs if you are not into this type of music.

Coloring books. This is another aspect of creative and imaginative play. After he has had the opportunity to color, it is a good idea to talk about what he has done. If you take one of his masterpieces and tack it up on the wall of his room, it will make him very happy and proud. While it hangs there it will serve as a constant reminder of his fine accomplishment.

Scrapbook. At this age your child can start putting together his own scrapbook by finding pictures in magazines and pasting them into his book. This can be an interesting project and should be all his own, although you will need to cut out the pictures (scissors and two- to three-year-olds don't mix). Such an activity is useful for developing feelings of independence.

Clay and Play-doh. These materials have already been taken up in the previous chapter. They remain excellent vehicles for your child to express his feelings through imaginative play. As he develops more strength and dexterity in his fingers, he will become more and more successful in creating all sorts of interesting shapes and objects.

Water play. Your child will continue to enjoy playing with and in water. You can supply him with some floating toys and let him splash around to his heart's content. Another interesting water-play activity requires a plastic straw and some soap flakes. You can then show him how to blow bubbles. This is a really sloppy activity, so I would suggest that after he is finished, you give him the chore of cleaning up the mess he is sure to have made. Again, never leave him alone near or in water.

Blackboard. Many parents do not think of this one. Buy a large blackboard that will give your child plenty of space to do his work. The best place to hang it is on a wall in his room. Supply him with pieces of different-colored chalk and he is in business. A blackboard is ideal for imaginative and creative drawing, and it also allows him to develop the skill of holding the chalk and manipulating it properly. This will make it easier for him to learn to handle pencils and pens, which will be such an important part of his armamentarium in school. I would suggest that you carefully explain to him that the chalk should only be used on the blackboard. Mrs. W. told me about her Alex, who had a lapse of memory about this instruction. Alex used his chalk to create a full-length mural covering the entire wall of his parents' newly painted bedroom.

Sharing. I have already explained that two- to three-year-olds are basically egocentric or self-centered. They are not very generous when it comes to sharing their possessions. While in the company of other children they play alongside rather than with them. Nevertheless, I believe that at this age sharing is an important concept for them to start to learn. The best time to teach your child about sharing is when there are other little children around. Get him used to the idea of sharing his toys with his friends. There will be much less trouble if you have enough toys for everybody. Explain that sharing is the right thing to do, and if he goes along with you, tell him how very happy his behavior has made you.

Silence. In *How to Parent,* Dr. Dodson describes an activity he calls the "silence game." This is good training for your child in terms of his schooling later on since it is designed to teach him to remain quiet and listen without talking – which is universally appreciated by teachers everywhere. To start with, tell him that you are about to play a game with him. This is very important because if he thinks it's a game he will pay attention to the instructions. Explain that the game is for both of you to sit quietly without saying a word and just listen for sounds. Then you say, "Now tell me what you hear." Try whispering an instruction to him or ask him to shut his eyes and tell you what noise you are making. Then you whistle or clap your hands or snap your fingers. I have suggested this game to many parents and they all tell me that it usually is a big success. Probably the best time to play it is shortly before reading your child his bedtime story, because it will serve to gradually quiet him down from his hard day of vigorous, noisy, stimulating activity.

T.V. I am including television in this section on emotional development to remind you how susceptible and vulnerable your little child is to what he sees and hears on the tube. I am referring particularly to television and violence. Many studies have shown that looking at violent T.V. programs is associated with increased aggressive behavior in a young child. The estimate is that the average child will see 18,000 T.V. murders by the time he finishes high school. As your child grows older it becomes more difficult for you to monitor his television watching. At this age, it should not be much of a problem. You must decide and control what programs your child watches. Observe how he reacts to what he sees on the television screen. If you notice that he gets too excited, confused, or upset, he is watching the wrong program and it should be turned off. This is not likely to happen if you have been selective and only allow him to watch one of the few excellent children's television programs, such as "Sesame Street" and "Blues Clues."

MENTAL (INTELLECTUAL) DEVELOPMENT

In the previous chapter I discussed the dangers of overburdening you child's mental capacities. I want to remind you again that too much of a good thing is just as bad as too little. Because of the competitive pressures of our society, many parents simply try too hard to raise a brighter child, a child who will be better able to handle the rigorous intellectual demands of our educational system. Since academic achievement is seen as a major indicator of success in our culture, many parents fall into the trap of trying too hard by attempting to teach their children more than they can handle. There is no scientific evidence proving that "stimulating" activities above and beyond the normal growth-promoting experiences we have been discussing lead in any way to advanced brain development.

Years ago the consensus was that good old common sense was all that was required to raise a child properly. We now believe that it takes more than that to give your child the best possible start. The entire thrust of this book has been to give you the added information and insight you need along with your own common sense to help make you the best possible parent. As I have done in each of the previous chapters, I will be offering you specific recommendations to help your child develop to his optimum intellectual potential. But before doing so, I want to caution you not to expect or demand too much too soon. How can a parent realize when he or she is pushing a child too hard? Probably the best way is by watching and listening to him. If he is happy with what you are doing together, you can rest assured that he is not being taxed beyond his mental capabilities. Stimulate and challenge his mind, but give him tasks at which he can succeed. Provide him with problem-solving situations that he can handle, and praise him each time he is successful. I believe that this is the ideal learning environment for a child and the best way to insure his subsequent success in school.

A few words about "problem based learning," a relatively new concept that many educators believe is a more effective way to teach than the old fashioned didactic method of just listening to somebody lecture and not actively participate. Many colleges and medical schools have switched from the straight lecture format to the problem-based approach with great success. So what does all this have to do with your toddler's learning? A whole lot. The concept of problem-based learning is based on making learning an adventure. The easiest way to understand problem-based learning is to think about it as a detective story. If you know who the murderer is on the first page it takes a lot of the mystery and fun out of the book. If your toddler is having fun learning, he will learn more quickly and retain more of what he has learned. Ask questions rather than lecturing to him. Give him simple problems to solve. The mother of almost three-year-old Sara proudly told me about how smart her daughter was. While on vacation Sara suffered a nasty sunburn (remember about sunscreens). Instead of telling her that the sun burned her, mama asked, "Why is your skin burned?" After a few seconds, with a big grin, Sara answered, "From hot sun." The lesson she learned will stick with her much longer because she figured it out for herself. Allow your child to think for himself. Of course, guide him in the right direction. Don't always be so quick with your answers. Rather, let him work out the problem by himself, if possible. When he succeeds he will be very proud of himself and will jump with joy, and so should you. Your role becomes less a lecturer and more a facilitator, a job that for many of us is more difficult, but this approach will help your child achieve his maximum intelligence potential.

Dr. Gessell, the famous child psychologist, uses the expression "word hungry" to describe the language development of the two- to three-year-old. This child is now anxious to learn more and more words, so any type of word game that you can think of will help satisfy his hunger for new words and new phrases. One of the keys to effective language acquisition is to play word games in which the child is asked questions about the world around him. It is clear that children learn language best in the context of their family life and you, the parents, act as the models they imitate. If you have a tendency to use baby talk, the result will be that your child will continue to use immature speech. It is important to use correct English when you talk to him. Ask and answer his questions without using baby talk. By doing so, you will more rapidly improve his primitive language. For example, if he says, "Where doggy is?" you can say, "Where is your dog? He is in the kitchen."

"Dr. Eden, Michael is driving me crazy," from a harassed mother. "He keeps asking me questions from morning until night. I feel guilty when I just don't have the time or strength to answer him." I assured her that it is both impossible and unnecessary to answer all his questions. There is no sense feeling guilty about this. All that can be expected of you is to do the best you can within the limits of your time and patience. When you do answer a question, make it short and simple. Your child is not interested in long, elaborate, detailed answers. Also, don't get upset if he asks the same question over and over again. Remember that his memory is far from perfect.

Your two- to three-year-old now realizes that everything has a name, and he wants to learn them all. You will notice that he will spend a great deal of time practicing words, just as he previously spent a great deal of his time practicing climbing up and down the stairs. When he correctly answers a question or learns a new word or new phrase, make certain that he knows you approve of his accomplishments. Besides asking him questions, another effective way of helping him learn language is to repeat thoughts frequently in different contexts. Let's use a toy car as an example. You can say, "Here is the car." Next time say, "Let's make the car run." You can then put the car away and say, "I don't see the car." Then bring the car back and run it along the floor, imitating the noise of the motor, and say, "The car makes a noise when it runs."

Above all, do not try to rush or push your child's speech development. Each child learns at his own individual pace. Make sure that your efforts to help him learn language remain fun. You can certainly help him develop language competence, but don't be frantic about it.

At this age, children often advance beyond just imitating and start to use what we call imaginative thinking skills. Whereas before he looked at and then handled play figures, he now starts to make these figures interact. He will pretend to put the baby figure to sleep or will move the baby figure to the mommy figure. He has figured out who these figures are and what they do, and plays with them appropriately. This type of thinking is a strong sign of intellectual growth.

By age three, many children will have a vocabulary of up to one thousand words and also will be able to put together a number of short, complex sentences. Often the child's language will be both imaginative and logical. There are times when his language will be more descriptive than your own. Two recent examples of this come to mind. A three-year-old who saw his bald-headed uncle come into the room pointed immediately to the bald scalp and said, "Skin-head." And a two-and-a-half-year-old who was playing in the park when a really obese lady came into view ran over to her and said at the top of his lungs, "Mommy, look at the big, round lady." Listen to your child carefully when he speaks. He may come up with some priceless sayings.

Many parents are overly concerned when their children mispronounce various sounds. By their third birthdays the majority of children make the following sounds correctly: mmm, nnn, ng, f, p, and h. They usually cannot as yet pronounce sss, sh, ch, wh, b, k, g, or r.

There is no reason to worry if your child cannot articulate certain sounds at this age. By the time he starts school his speech pattern will be greatly improved. If you have any questions about how his speech is developing, consult your child's doctor.

SPECIFIC SUGGESTIONS

The following are specific suggestions and recommendations to help your child develop his intellectual capabilities to the fullest.

Jigsaw puzzles. Simple jigsaw puzzles without too many different pieces are readily available. These are usually made out of wood or sturdy plastic. Jigsaw puzzles are challenging to your child and enjoyable for him to solve. Besides complimenting him when he puts one together, talk to him about the object that the completed puzzle represents.

Clay and Play-doh. I have included these in this section because they can help your child in his language development. Words such as top, side, flat, round, smooth, and rough should be used when you talk to him about what he has created.

Crayons and pencils. Supply your child with large sheets of paper and a good-sized crayon or pencil. Most two- to three-year-olds spend happy times scribbling away, and this is good practice for their future writing and drawing. These little children are very proud of what they have "written" on the paper, so when your child brings his handiwork to you for approval, tell him what a good job he has done. There will be times when, with some imagination on your part, you may be able to pick out a specific object that he unintentionally drew on the scribbled page. If this occurs, show it to him and talk to him about it. He may try to do it again but it's unlikely that he will succeed.

Instructions. At this age your child's mind is sophisticated enough to follow more than one instruction at a time. He can understand and remember rather complicated directions. Instead of simply asking him to do one particular chore and then, after he has completed it, to do another, give him a bigger challenge. For example, "Please go to your room and bring back your toy teddy and then put it on the sofa." Your child may get it right the first time, but if he mixes up the directions, repeat the same set of instructions, of course without showing anger or disappointment. When he succeeds, celebrate his accomplishment with a big hug and tell him how well he has done.

Bedtime ritual. This is a must not only in terms of your child's emotional security, but also for learning. Children look forward to the bedtime routine and it is an ideal way to end each of their days. To help your little child wind down and prepare for sleep, eliminate roughhouse activities and television watching before bedtime. More appropriate activities are taking a bath, eating a snack, and finally reading a story while he is tucked into bed. Read him a story appropriate for his age that he is interested in. Show him the pictures and ask him questions about what you are reading. As an alternative, you can make up your own story. I remember a running serial that I continued for months on end when our son was this age. He would remind me where I stopped the night before if I forgot and started off in the wrong place.

Trips. Take advantage of your child's inexhaustible zest for new experiences by taking him out on as many trips as you possibly can. These trips expand his horizons and stimulate his brain, and are important in helping him learn while having a good time. I am referring to trips to the zoo, library, or museum. Take him to the firehouse and to construction sites so that he can watch and learn about people working. There is also nothing wrong with taking him out to eat. It is surprising how well-behaved most two- or three-year-olds are in a restaurant. I would hesitate to pick an elegant, expensive French restaurant as his first experience, but there is certainly no reason to automatically assume that your child will only enjoy one of the fast-food establishments.

Children's records and tapes. Many excellent children's records and tapes are now available and these are certainly good vehicles for learning.

Children's books with pictures. I have already referred to these as they relate to the bedtime ritual. Obviously, children should be read to at other times as well. The more books in the house, the better. One of the major cornerstones of your child's learning is your reading and explaining and asking questions about what you have read. These reading sessions should stop at the first sign of boredom or disinterest. Try to read aloud stories that have a range of characters and situations. This encourages creative thinking, a key to intellectual development. As your toddler approaches his third birthday, he should be ready to start going to the library and a library card of his own is a great birthday present. Let me repeat that reading literacy is the key to success in school.

Television. In terms of your child's intellectual development television may play a useful role only if used sensibly. However, it usually works the other way around. Your job is to find the appropriate T.V. children's programs for him to watch and not allow him to waste many hours looking at cartoons or programs filled with violence. When possible, watch these programs along with your child and ask him to try some of the activities he sees. He will learn much more if you are there to answer his questions and stimulate his interest. However, limit T.V. watching to a maximum of one to two hours per day. A University of Washington in Seattle study published in 2005 compared the amount of television watching before age three with performance on three nationally recognized reading tests at ages six and seven. It turned out that "each hour of daily T.V. viewing before age three was associated with deleterious effects." The great majority of these T.V. hours were spent watching cartoons. The bottom line is that excessive T.V. watching for two- to three-year-olds results in dumber (and fatter) children. A final word about T.V. and how it is currently affecting our children's lives: A large-scale survey of the homes of preschool-age children showed that two-thirds had a T.V. in their bedroom, and one-half had a T.V. in the kitchen or dining room. T.V. watching is taking up too much time that could be much better spent reading or playing.

Computers and videogames. There is plenty of time for your little child to become a computer programmer and a whiz at videogames. For now I would suggest you stick to books. With older siblings in the house, it is more difficult to keep your toddler away from the videogames. My advice is to discourage your toddler by distracting him and by convincing his older brother or sister to keep the games away from him. The consensus among experts in the field is that neither videogames nor computers have much of a role in helping a toddler learn much of anything. I have a real problem with the video games that are full of violent action and the amount of time children spend playing with them. A number of studies involving school-age children and teenagers have demonstrated a correlation between violent game action and violent behavior. I am not aware of such studies with two- to three-year olds, but it makes intuitive sense to believe the same would hold true for toddlers. But even if this type of videogame doesn't lead to violence in two- to three-year-olds, it certainly doesn't help your child develop to his maximum potential. And so the bottom line is that these videogames are either damaging or a waste of time, and either way they should not be a part of your toddler's life.

Educational toys. There is a tremendous and ever-growing industry out there, the "educational toy" business. Certainly, parents want to give their young children every edge possible to encourage their intellectual development. Reading and hearing about all the miraculous advances these toys can provide makes it difficult for parents not to jump on the bandwagon. I am asked about "Baby Mozart" at least once a week. If some of these toys do not interfere with what I have advised you to do throughout Positive Parenting and with a lot of more important stuff, such as dancing and wrestling with your child, be my guest. But I don't really believe that educational toys play much of a role in your child's development during these first three years of life and most other authorities in the field agree with me. They might be helpful as long as they are not used to excess, but the claims from the manufacturers often are overstated and there is no proof of their accuracy. While these toys seem to have no negative effects on your child, there has been no proof that they have any benefits.

Word games. I referred to word games in the introduction to this chapter. Since our two- to three-year-old is so anxious to learn new words and phrases, he will be more than ready for this type of activity. For example, point to a ball and say, "I see something round. What it is?" or say, "It's cold today. What should we wear when we go out?" The possibilities for these word-game activities are endless, and they do much to develop and enhance your child's language and thinking skills.

Self-correction. You can indirectly teach your child that it is acceptable for him to make mistakes without worrying too much about them. This is an interesting concept and makes a good deal of sense, provided you don't do it too often or make a game of it. For example, you can say, "Where is 'poon?" "No, not 'poon. Where is spoon?" If he sees that you are not infallible, it will be easier for him to practice his language and not be overly concerned about the mistakes he makes. Again, rather than criticizing him when he is wrong, correct him instead.

Conversation and discussion. Between two and three years of age, two-way conversation between you and your child is still rather limited. Nonetheless, it is extremely important that you talk with him rather than just give orders. Listen to him talk and take turns talking. Teach him as you talk together. For example, if he says, "See doggy," you say, "Yes, I see the dog. He barks." He will often mix up the word order. You should correct him by then saying the words in their correct order. It is not necessary to always ask him to repeat it correctly. He will learn for himself in time.

Mealtimes should be used for discussion. Too few families regularly sit down to eat together around the table. I encourage you to do so whenever possible. Meals should not be eaten watching T.V. or reading a newspaper. This is the ideal time to ask your child about what he has done and seen that day. Give him the chance to talk about his experiences as best he can. Rather than trying to keep him quiet so that he can concentrate on eating, allow him to be more of an active participant in mealtime conversations. Talking together like this has been shown to be a positive factor in school achievement.

MYTH: In order to be a positive parent, you must be highly educated and you must supply your child with all sorts of elaborate, expensive equipment and toys.

Wrong on both counts. If you have read through this book, it should be obvious that you do not need a great deal of formal education, nor do you need to buy lots of fancy games, materials, and equipment.

Let me end our journey through the wondrous first three years of your child's life with the following reminder: most child-development experts, including me, consider sterile tools such as flash cards, Mozart CDs, computer games, and television less effective than more social and emotional interactive activities, such as reading to or talking to your child. The best way to maximize your child's intelligence potential is to develop a loving and trusting relationship with him, and the earlier, the better. You do this by interacting with him – kissing, hugging, tickling, wrestling, laughing, and reading together. Play with him and tell him you love him every single day and you will do fine. It is as simple as that.

I hope that I have given you some insights into what goes on during your child's first three years and what you can do to help him grow up healthier, happier, and smarter.

Happy third birthday!

Epilogue

THE TWELVE COMMANDMENTS OF POSITIVE PARENTING

It is obvious that Positive Parenting does not stop at age three. Your job is just beginning. If you have given your child the best that's in you up to now, she is well on her way toward becoming what you hope for – a responsible, successful, loving, happy adult. But even if you haven't been the most Positive Parent so far, it's not too late to start.

1. Challenge and stimulate the mind.
2. Overburdening must be avoided
3. Make it easy for curiosity and independence to flourish.
4. Make certain that you set proper examples.
5. Admire and build up your child's self-esteem.
6. Never hit or abuse in anger.
7. Don't set unrealistic goals.
8. Make available the proper tools, activities, space, and opportunities.
9. Encourage exercise and physical fitness and a nutritious diet.
10. Nurture them with love and laughter.
11. Trust them.
12. Spend "quality time" together.

There is still plenty of time to get it right and the sooner you start, the better. Positive Parenting never ends, no matter the age of your child. And down the road, if you are fortunate enough to be blessed with grandchildren, your parenting journey will continue. But now it will be called "Positive

Grandparenting." Come to think of it, that's a pretty good title for my next book. Your goal remains the same as it has been from the start – to raise the healthiest, happiest, and smartest child possible. I believe that your chances for success increase if you continue to follow the Twelve Commandments of Positive Parenting.

Good Luck and Happy Positive Parenting!

Index